Patricia –
Enjoy and
God Bless
Alberta H. Sequ—
2008

A Healing Heart
A Spiritual Renewal

By Alberta Sequeira

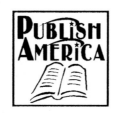

PublishAmerica
Baltimore

ISBN: 1-4241-4458-2

PUBLISHED BY PUBLISHAMERICA, LLLP

www.publishamerica.com

Baltimore

Printed in the United States of America

In Memory of my Father,
Brigadier General, Albert L. Gramm, Sr.

Dedicated to the Gramm Family...
Our Beloved Mother: Sophie Gramm
Children: Leona, Walter, (deceased), Albert, Alberta, Bill, Joe
Grandchildren: Debbie, Lori, David, Danny, Brandon, Olivia, Molly
Great Grandchildren: Kerri, Michael, Joe, Meagan, Joshua, Elizabeth
To our husbands and wives who have blessed our family:
Bob, Maria, Al, Sharon, Marge, Brian, Andrea

Acknowledgments

I will place my law within them, and write it upon their hearts; I will be their God, and they shall be my people. Jeremiah 31:33

A Healing Heart contains my thoughts and beliefs and is, I hope, a witness to the actions of God in our lives. This journey would not have happened if I had not responded to Him. It was through the silence that I had opened my heart to listen.

I am indebted to all who had supported me through my years working on this book. First, I want to thank my family, who understood my desire to leave the military status of my father to our grandchildren and, hopefully, future generations of the Gramm family.

This book is dedicated to my beloved father, who had more of himself to be explored than I had realized. I'm grateful for his teachings of the importance of family; faith in God, and for his guidance in my growing years.

I give my deepest love to my husband, Al, who lifted me when I had lost confidence and gave me the strength to go on.

I'm forever grateful to my brother, Joe, for all his hard work and devoted attention in the modification to the pictures and for his help in retrieving the military information on our father.

I'm thankful for my dearest friends, Arlene Albert of Vero Beach, Florida, and Eddie Sousa of West Warwick, Rhode Island for their years of encouragement and faith in seeing my book in print.

Many thanks go to my editor, Jerine Watson, and my co-editor, Steven Manchester, for their guidance of my writing, and Darcie Roy, for her talent in my final editing.

I'm indebted to Greg Sousa, the photographer, who had sat for an hour on a pier in Sanibel Island, Florida, and captured the incredible picture for my book cover. Greg lives in Ft. Myers, Florida.

A heartfelt appreciation of my writer's group in Dartmouth, Massachusetts for their critiques that made this happen.

A sincere admiration to the comrades of the 26th Yankee Division, who fought with my father during WWII, and of his many personal friends, who had supplied information on the battles in France and Germany:

Retired Lieutenant Colonel Fred N. Kawa, of Whitman, Massachusetts; Joe Devine of North Weymouth, Massachusetts (26th Yankee Division, 101st Infantry, Company B); James C. Haahr, Author of *The Command is Forward; the 101st Infantry in Lorraine* (26th Yankee Division, 101st Infantry, Company C); Jim Neville, Curator of Camp Drum, New York; Dennis J. O"Brien, of Fort Myers, Florida (26th Yankee Division, 104th Infantry, Company G); Bernard Huntley of Rockland, Massachusetts (26th Yankee Division); Richard I. Paul, of Destin, Florida, retired LTC US Army, (26th Yankee Division).

Introduction

As a child, I prayed with confidence and faith; nothing was impossible with God.

As the years passed, and I got older, I looked at life differently with its hardships and disappointments.

Life became a reality with sadness from losing a parent, friends, and surviving a shattered marriage.

My confidence turned to doubt and my faith weakened.

I wondered where God was when my prayers went unanswered.

I had to remind myself that no matter how hard things were, God always answers our prayers.

It will be in His time, will, and way.

Birth, life, and death are stages we travel through until we return once again, to Our Maker.

We must never give up praying, for if we do, we will not return to our faith or receive the many gifts and graces that await us. We must pray, not only to survive, but so we can unite and come closer to God.

—Alberta H. Sequeira

Chapter 1
Miracles Around Us

"Dad, do you believe in miracles?"

He turned, looking at me with a shocked expression on his face, "Of course I do. Don't you?"

It was a question he probably never expected a daughter in her forties to be asking him. With our strong religious upbringing, I could see he was stunned for a second with my asking.

"Yes, I do, Dad, but I wish we lived in the times when God was on earth and we witnessed Him heal with our own eyes," I answered.

He gave me a loving but disappointed look and then turned to put down the books he was carrying. Slowly, he placed them back into the living room bookshelves he had just polished. He had built the unit for my mother a few years back.

Once he completed the task, he explained, "Honey, there are miracles around us each and every day. We just don't take the time to see them. People are healed from terminal diseases when doctors had given them no hope, or a person walked when they were told it would be impossible. You can witness a mystical event without ever knowing how it happened. No one stops to realize these are miracles and that they come from God. You need to look, listen and watch more closely to things around you."

We shared this talk on a beautiful, hot summer day back in June of

1986. It was one of my many visits to my parents' home in East Falmouth, Massachusetts. Having had this personal conversation with my father, made me realize how unusual it had been. Our discussions, often than not, were amongst other family members.

The sun was shining directly through the large bay window in the living room and I could feel the warmth of it going through me as we stood there talking. I took life with my father for granted, never realizing time was disappearing and the moments left with him were counting down.

He was always in good health and very active at seventy-six years old. Dad was not one for sitting around in front of television all day. If Mom did not have things for him to fix, he would find projects on his own to keep busy. It took him months to build a beautiful fieldstone fireplace all by himself in the back yard. He completed replacing and installing all the storm windows for their low level ranch home, and took pride with keeping the yard in flawless condition.

Albert L. Gramm, Sr. was a proud and distinguished retired Brigadier General, but to his children, he was just our father. He still had a solid physique and loved showing his strong, firm legs when he wore his summer shorts. Every outfit was matched and he never went anywhere without wearing one of the Cape Cod hats from his collection. He tried to hide his thinning gray hair by combing it to the side, giving it the impression of being thicker.

Dad was always a hard person for me to get close to because he never showed his emotions. He was a man of very few words. My father demonstrated his feelings by never failing to give me a warm smile along with a wink when he passed by me, going from one project to another. One small gesture, and yet it made me feel so loved.

I acted no differently than him when it came to opening about how bad things really were during my marriage and after my divorce. These troubles were locked deep within and I never asked for help or advice from my parents.

Divorced and on my own, decisions were always facing me. I didn't want to throw any turmoil my parents' way. My four siblings often looked to Dad for advice on important matters. It was something that I

8

routinely omitted to do. I had felt that if I was old enough to get married, I was old enough to handle my own problems.

I had three brothers, Albert (my twin), Bill, Joe and a sister, Leona. We ranged in age from our thirties to fifties, though Mom often remarked, "You'll always be kids to Dad and I no matter how old you all get."

In 1944, we had a brother, Walter, who died at seven years old from Polio. It affected Leona as well as my parents, for years. Leona had been a year older and they had done everything together.

I avoided the thought of Dad not being in my life. When the death of a loved one comes unexpectedly, or even with warning, we're still not as prepared as we think. When we receive news that someone we know has passed away, our heart goes out to the family left behind facing their heartbreak. After attending the funeral and sharing in their loss, we all go right back to our responsibilities with no distraction or upset in our daily routine.

The impact of death does not truly affect someone emotionally until it hits us personally. This is when we face how unfair and devastating the loss is. Our world comes to a complete stop from the reality of it— we are immobilized.

It's now October of 1990 as I sit in a rocking chair facing my father lying in bed, dying of cancer. He now needs a miracle like the one we talked about so long ago.

I had thought the death of either parent would be far distant, years from now. Mom was seventy-six and her mother was still living at ninety-five. Dad's father died of cancer in his late seventies but our father came across strong as a horse, never having any serious illness. The reality of his cancer was catching up with me and there was little time left to know about his life: not only as a father, but just as a person.

I wondered, how I had allowed all my years to go by, without ever caring to learn who he was, and what he was all about. Who was he really besides a father, husband, and one who worked hard every day to support his family? He had to have had dreams. We all do.

I prayed as I watched him, asking God to help me find a way to heal my heart from being so selfish with my own wants and needs.

Chapter 2
Family Members

During my growing years at home, every morning I watched Dad leave the house for work, always remembering to kiss my mother goodbye. The same ritual would be performed upon his return after a hard day. I took no time to ask him what he did in his career. I knew he joined the National Guard in 1928 and served in the Army during WWII and held the title of Brigadier General at his retirement. I didn't know the history he carried throughout his lifetime.

It was rare when weekends at our house were not filled with laughter from my parents' friends. Many of the men served with Dad during the war. Every few months, the couples would take turns entertaining at their own home. Their service years were the loud topics that went around the kitchen table while the couples played cards. That was the time I should have been within listening distance to hear and learn what their lives were all about when they were young. With the devastating casualties during wartime, it was a blessing from God that our father came home alive and unharmed.

A new world had opened up for me after ending my fourteen-year marriage. I felt very independent and proud to handle all my problems without asking my parents for any help. The tension dropped when I was able to make decisions with my own life and my daughters. The sad part was that I still loved my ex-husband. Before his drinking got out of hand, he was a very gentle and loving person.

The stress in our marriage had me on the verge of a breakdown. I had spent the last four years in private counseling and two month of sessions with my husband in the Alcoholic Anonymous program. He told his counselor he did not have a drinking problem and decided to stop his meetings. With no hope from his denial, I divorced him to keep myself together.

It wasn't until he had been hospitalized that he admitted to me that his drinking was killing him. It was sad when he wanted to change his life and it was too late. On February 10, 1985, he died from cirrhosis of the liver at the early age of forty-five.

I lived an hour away from my parents home, so I wasn't available, as often as I should've been, to help my father when he first got sick. At the time, Dad was going back and forth to the doctor's office because of discomfort under his right rib. We all thought it was just something minor and it caused no major concern to any of us.

Between my brothers, my sister, and I, one of us was available to help out when it was necessary. We all lived in Massachusetts and an hour was the longest for any of us to arrive at their house. My brother, Joe, and his wife, Marge, lived in Yarmouth, so they visited our parents frequently to see how they were doing. Their business, Gramm Upholstery, kept them busy but they could take time off whenever there was a need. They were both very active and loved any outdoor sports; especially canoeing or camping.

Leona and, her husband, Bob, lived in Buzzard Bay and owned the Waltman Lumber Outlet in Wareham. Leona stayed in touch with Dad on a daily basis and took him on his numerous doctor appointments. They both worked everyday at the lumberyard, except Wednesdays, so rarely did they have time to themselves.

My twin brother, Albert, and his wife, Maria, lived in Stoughton and dropped by on the weekends because they both had a business to run. Maria owned a hair salon in Norwood with her two sisters, Diane and Lisa. It was named Dante's III after their father and the numeral number stood for the three daughters. Albert was running his company, Gramm

Sign, from their home. He made outside commercial business signs and any that had been requested for a business office.

Dante and Carmela Picciano, Maria's parents, had bought a lot behind my parents' house and had built a beautiful home there. It was wonderful having the two families get together for cookouts or just everyday visits.

My brother, Bill, and his wife, Sharon, lived in Scituate and squeezed visits in between their busy schedules. Bill worked for Leona at the Waltman Lumber Outlet as the company's Yard Manager. Sharon worked for a catering business that frequently serviced President John F. Kennedy's family at their compound in Hyannisport. They did most of the Kennedy's events and we all loved listening to her talk about the famous stars that attended.

Our parents were home most of the time and no one worried about the formality of calling first. The ride was always enjoyable because of the beautiful scenery along the Cape, so it was never a wasted trip, if they weren't home.

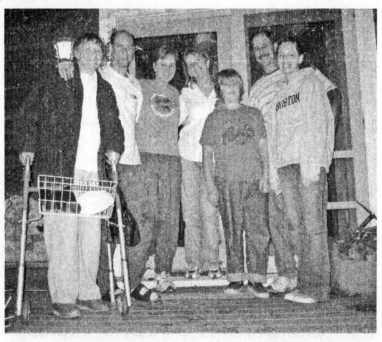

Left to right: Mom, Joe, Marge, Sharon, Brandon, Bill, Olivia

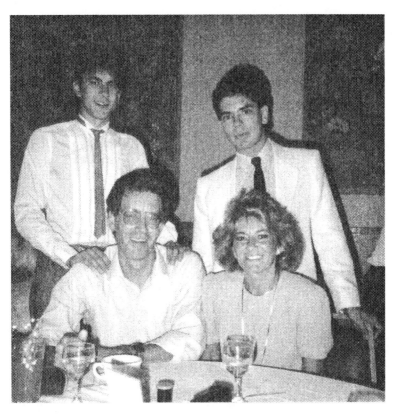

Back left: Dan & David: Front left: Albert & Maria

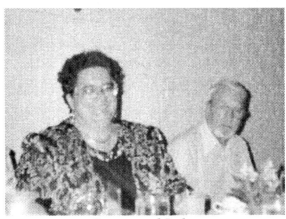

Leona and Bob

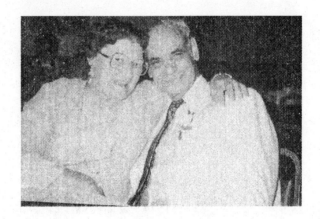

Mom and Dad

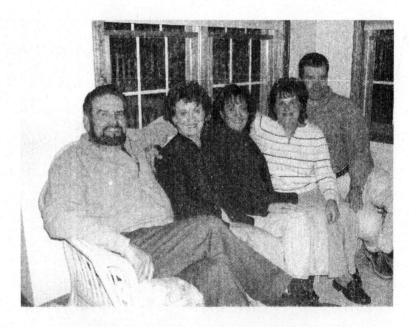

Left: Al, Alberta, Lori, Debbie & Brian

Chapter 3
The Beginning of the End

In 1988, Dad had surgery for cancer of the prostate at the Falmouth Hospital. After the procedure, the urologist informed him there was a small amount of cancer left behind. Because this particular type of cancer was very slow moving, his doctor thought it could be controlled if it had spread by Dad's next physical. He sent Dad home telling him not to worry about it.

The family begged our father to go to a hospital in Boston for a second opinion, but he had complete faith in his doctor. He insisted no further tests were going to be done, unless they were ordered by his doctor. No amount of talking or pleading could change his mind.

We all feared his condition was serious. He still kept up with chores including: painting the house, mowing the lawn and any other maintenance. Dad always accomplished anything that had to be done. He still tackled new projects to keep active, even though he had slowed down with age.

It was eight months after the prostate surgery when my father started to experience the pain on his right side. Leona had had gallbladder surgery in the past and Dad spoke to her about his symptoms thinking he might have the same problem.

I telephoned Dad frequently after he called me himself and informed me about his tests. He assured me he would call when the results came back from the doctor. In addition to his illness, we also spoke about some medical problems I was having: There was the possibility of me going into the hospital sometime in the future for surgery to remove fibroid tumors from my uterus.

Weeks went by and I hadn't heard anything, so I called him. He insisted everything was fine and that he was still waiting for all the test results.

Meanwhile, the rest of the family met at Albert and Maria's house to make arrangements for a surprise birthday party for both my parents. Joe had suggested the Roadside Café in Hyannis since he'd been there before. He said they had a large menu and everyone would have a good choice to choose from it. Dad's birthday fell on March 27th and Mom's was the 28th so we always combined the celebration, but, this was the first really big party to commemorate their birthdays.

I invited my boyfriend, Al, of four years' duration, to join us. We arrived at the restaurant to find the back room had already been decorated with pink and blue balloons. They hung over two long tables, with flower centerpieces on each table. Gradually the room filled with my brothers and their wives, my sister and her husband, and the grandkids David, Dan, Lori, and Debbie with her husband Brian. Dante and Carmela Picciano came to share in the event.

Dad and Mom entered the doorway with no surprised reactions on their faces; which I found odd and disappointing. I figured that someone must have tipped them off about the party before arriving. Once everyone gave them a hug and kiss, they went immediately to their seats and settled at one of the tables. As the room started to echo with deafening laughter and the noise of mixed conversations, neither of them made any movement to join in the chaos.

When Leona walked towards to me, I took her arm and pulled her aside asking if anything was wrong with them. She whispered that Dad had told her that morning that the test results showed his cancer had spread to his stomach and liver. My parents were devastated. *God this can't be happening.*

What a terrible day for them to be under more stress with a surprise party. I suddenly felt sick, but kept my emotions to myself. I didn't know who else knew and was not about to say anything. It would only make my parents feel worse if the results spread.

Our father was turning eighty and it was a big moment for the family. The two waitresses placed the menus on the tables as we all squeezed together elbow to elbow.

My sister-in-law, Sharon, abruptly stood up raising her wine glass. The rest of us followed her action. Looking directly at Dad and Mom, with the warmest and most loving smile, she replied, "Happy birthday to both of you! May you enjoy and share in many, many more wonderful years together. We love you."

The room filled with applause as we shouted with approval from Sharon's toast. I assumed she was not aware of the situation as she was very natural without tears. Dad and Mom stared back with unfamiliar forced smiles on their faces.

After dinner, the waitresses then brought out two large cakes lit with candles and all of them joined right in with us singing "Happy Birthday."

We all had enjoyed planning the party for my parents but they were probably glad when the evening ended. Their minds could not have been focused on the celebration. The happy and secure world they were living in had just collapsed.

Dad was now fighting an aggressive stomach and liver cancer less than a year after his prostate surgery. The one his doctor told him not to worry about because it metastasized slowly! I couldn't help being bitter and wondered if it could've been cured if they had done further testing right after the surgery. They might have discovered that it had spread to the other organs which it obviously had done.

Chapter 4
Dad's Surgery

Leona stayed at my parent's house the night before Dad's surgery. They both shared a large bowl of grapes, and after consuming half of them, Dad had had agonizing stomach pain. It never occurred to either of them what the acid would do to the ulceration in his stomach. My sister thought he would have to be taken to the hospital before morning, but my father suffered through the throbbing discomfort until it subsided.

On April, 25, 1990, Dad's surgery was performed at the South Shore Hospital in Weymouth. Family members filled the waiting room. A nurse came to informed us that we would be notified of his condition when the surgery was done. In the meantime, we tried to occupy our minds by reading the magazines placed on the corner tables. It was impossible to concentrate, so we headed for the cafeteria to get something to eat.

A few hours later, we headed back to the waiting room. When the procedure was completed, we saw Dad being wheeled from the operating room towards Recovery. We all clapped and waved to him as they took him down the hall. As he was wheeled by, he gave a groggy stare in our direction.

Once he was comfortable in Recovery, Mom was allowed to visit him. After fifteen minutes, she came down the hall toward us, smiling. She jumped straight up in the air and slapped her two feet together like a professional dancer. How she did that at seventy-six was beyond me. Our hearts jumped, too, with hope.

My mother informed us he had seventy percent of his stomach removed. When Dad saw her, even with strong medication, he immediately said, "Oh, Sophie, the pain is awful." The thought of him suffering that much was like a knife going through my heart. I left the hospital feeling he was in good hands.

The next day we arrived at the hospital to take turns visiting Dad. When Albert and Maria entered the waiting room, I noticed Maria didn't seem like herself and had an additional aura of sadness about her, over and above our father's condition. When Albert went in to see Dad, she suddenly whispered, "Albert went to the doctor's office yesterday and it's not good news."

Albert had been experiencing what he thought was a bad cold leaving him with an unusually deep, scratchy voice that wasn't normal. When he spoke, it was very hard to understand what he was saying. It sounded like a real bad case of laryngitis. My brother was in his forties but had been a very heavy smoker since he was a teenager.

His primary doctor told him it was bronchitis. Months later, he strained his voice when he spoke and he was hoarse. He went to another doctor for a second opinion. The diagnosis was throat cancer.

Oh, Lord, no! The news almost brought me to my knees. I felt the news go right through me, since we were twins. Albert was going to be faced with a hard, painful road ahead of him. Here it was the day after Dad's cancer surgery and Albert was now in the same situation facing a similar life-threatening disease. How were my parents going to handle this?

Dad was allowed two visitors at a time for a short period. In addition to the pain from surgery, he was also fighting a fibrillation problem in his heart. This was something he had dealt with since his late twenties. They were trying to find a medication to control the irregular heartbeat.

It was easy for Albert and me to understand his heart problem. We both had had streptococcus numerous times when we were young and developed rheumatic fever from it. Because of this, we had to have our tonsils out and were admitted into a hospital for three months. This caused us to develop heart disease and have had episodes of fibrillation most of our lives. Both of us are still taking different medications for this problem.

When my turn came to visit my father, I was amazed to see how good he looked after his ordeal. He was sitting up and talking to the nurses like he was in complete charge of his arrhythmia, advising them which medications to give him. Through the years, he knew which ones controlled his fast heart rate. His problem continued for several weeks.

I sat down in the chair next to him and overheard Albert talking to him about his own cancer. They were both discussing it with controlled emotions. Albert explained a doctor from the Boston Medical Center had offered to do an experimental radiation procedure that had never been used on anyone before. He had already signed up to be their first patient. My brother and father discussed every avenue to take with both their treatments which would be done at the same time; Albert with radiation and Dad with chemo.

I found myself at a loss for words, trying to make conversation with my father and felt uncomfortable because of it. Albert helped the situation by staying in the room but it made me realize how little time I had spent in conversations with Dad.

I was aware of the strong love our father had for all of us. Sitting there with nothing to say, made me wonder why I should be feeling this way in his presence. Now and then I would say something insignificant to blend into the topics going back and forth between the two of them. After my visiting time was up, I left to go home feeling empty inside.

Chapter 5
The Absent Communication

Since there was a half hour drive facing me to get home, it gave me time to analyze why there was always a distancing feeling with my father through the years.

I remembered back, before Dad's diagnosis, to a moment when after a visit at my parent's house in East Falmouth, I was leaving to go home with Debbie and Lori. While I was hugging my father goodbye, I had a desire to hold onto him a little longer than usual. There was no particular reason, except a sudden need to feel close after having spent a nice day with him.

My father must have felt uncomfortable because he stopped hugging me first and stepped back. I smiled and embraced him again, explaining I wanted a special hug. He allowed me that but he seemed stiff. Our hugs were always very fast and I don't think he knew how to handle this odd request.

My father's routine of saying goodbye to anyone was to go outside and stand at the end of the driveway and wave. It could be in the dead of winter and snowing, and he would never fail to put his coat and boots on to stand out there. His hand would be high in the air along with a warm smile on his face. He wouldn't go back inside the house until we were out of sight.

The children and grandchildren grew to know this ritual and

participated in the farewell ritual at each departure: we in turn would wave until the car turned the corner.

Thinking back to this made me realize there was a soft side to Dad. Some men have no trouble expressing their feelings openly. My father would hide his emotions behind the action of helping with our personal hardships or financial problems. My mother had remarked once that our father took command of his family the way he did with the military men who served under him, by making decisions. He wanted to be in control of every situation.

I thought back when I was seven years old and my father and I would share special moments living at my childhood house in West Springfield. He loved watching boxing and the program *Victory At Sea* whenever they were on television.

I would slowly edge my way over to where Dad was sitting. My desire was not to be on his lap or have a conversation with him. My goal was to sit on the floor facing the television, lean my back against his chair and wrap both my arms around his lower legs. There I would sit and watch the program, with absolutely no interest in it, only sharing the time with him.

My father would sit and smoke his pipe, and how I loved the smell of it! He would place his hand on top of my head gently and rub it slowly as he watched his favorite shows. There was no talking between us, just the gentle sentiment of affection.

After my divorce, my father wanted to help me by giving a down payment for a used car. I swallowed my pride and decided to take his offer. He started to car hunt in the Falmouth area and I did the same in my surrounding locations.

This was how I met my future husband, Al Sequeira. He was a manager of a Taunton dealership I visited. As I pulled into the lot, I noticed him in my rearview mirror, walking toward me.

Once he came upon me, I became aware of how well dressed and business-like he was. His attire consisted of light gray dress pants and a dark navy sport jacket. Al's appearance caught my eye right away along with his masculine good looks. His black wavy hair had a touch of gray along with his close-trimmed beard and mustache.

His taste in clothes showed his self-confidence and his smile melted my heart. Al didn't come across as being pushy with his sales pitch but was very informative and experienced in the car business. I didn't end up purchasing a car through him only because my father found a Ford Escort that I loved at another dealership.

God works in strange ways, putting people in our paths for bigger and better things. Because of my father's offer to help me, I went out to search for a car and instead found a lasting friendship and romance with Al.

Now, looking back, I realized Dad had always been there for me to develop an open relationship with him. The feeling of distance was mine: not inviting my father into my life and not trying to enter his. Now, I know the importance of not only talking to a person but listening, if you want to know them.

There was so much Dad didn't know about me. I tried to show how independent I was by doing everything myself, including repairs to my own home. The doors to communication between us were shut because I never asked for help when I needed it. I thought asking for assistance was sign of weakness. But what did I gain from it?

All those visits to see my parents throughout my lifetime consisted of superficial talks. Dad would asked, "How are you?"

"Good," I would reply.

"How are the girls?"

"They're both busy with school and friends," I would answer not getting into any real problems.

No honesty was ever displayed to my parents. They should have been told the truth that I was doing awful. Why was I afraid to admit that the bills were piling up and the girls were struggling emotionally from their parents' divorce? I started to understand that hidden problems wouldn't go away.

How would I feel if my daughters were struggling and did not tell me? I hoped this wrong action would not pass down to my daughters' way of thinking. They never saw their mother cry or show the weakness of the fear of being alone. I hid my feelings from them, when I had been struggling to keep the family together. How could someone get to know me when I hid everything from everyone? I never really sat and talked to my daughters to learn what they're feeling. I could not deal with emotions at that time. I wanted to keep the girls' lives as normal as possible.

These were my thoughts and conclusions as I drove home from the hospital, wondering why I had nothing to say to my father. His having cancer and being operated on was probably the most I knew about him. If we were close, maybe he would've told me how he was actually doing mentally and physically with the disease. I never asked. Instead, I sat there depending completely on Albert to carry the whole conversation so I could just smile when Dad looked at me. He and I never conversed and I envied my brother for being so close to our father.

Why couldn't I ask him how he was doing? Was I afraid of hearing he might be scared of not being cured and dying?

This was the first time that I took the time to study my relationship with my father. I'd misjudged him. I truly believed Dad was doing it all wrong, when it had actually been me. I don't ever remember, sitting alone with my father and having any private conversations on any topic. I avoided the intimacy. I am not sure why this happened.

When I was young, my mother had a breakdown after giving birth to my brother, Joe. Mom had a hard time dealing with her own emotions. Being young, I sensed that something was wrong, and kept my distance from her. Now I realized that I didn't open myself up to my parents even back then. This could've been a habit that I carried growing up.

Chapter 6
Facing Mortality

Al and I decided to make a trip to visit my parents one Sunday afternoon. Once we arrived, the two of us joined the family that had congregated around the kitchen table. They were all talking to Mom about Dad's condition. In the meantime, my father was sitting in an armchair in the living room watching television.

Al and I went to join him so he wouldn't be alone. Entering the room, we found him hanging off the seat. I'll never forget the sight. He was on his back with his head forward, causing his chin to be bent against his chest with his buttocks hanging off the seat. He was only balanced by his elbows and waist leaning into the bottom edge of the chair cushion to keep him off the floor.

Together we gently lifted him under his arms and placed him back into the chair in a straight-up sitting position.

He looked up at us, and said in a tremendously frail voice, "I've never felt so weak in my entire life."

His remark went right through me. He hadn't had the strength to call out to anyone.

Dad had received his chemo treatments a few weeks after his surgery. Leona told me the thought of having the procedure frightened him so much that he couldn't keep the first appointment, and had to reschedule. Our father had faced everything head on in life-except this disease. It had weakened all his muscles; leaving him helpless to get around anywhere.

I couldn't imagine what he was experiencing physically and emotionally. It had to be indescribable. No matter how many people were around him, he had probably felt alone. The expression, "We enter this world alone, and we leave it alone," is so true.

Watching my father in this slow, painful progression and not being able to do anything for him was a nightmare that was becoming unbearable. Day after day, this incurable disease was sucking the life out of him. I started to appreciate how precious life is and what an irreplaceable gift it is from God.

Witnessing how death was attacking his body and mind, scared me into facing my own mortality, which I was not comfortable doing.

I had gone through similar emotions a few years earlier when my girlfriend, Sandy, passed away from cancer. For years, we were close friends, until I started to slowly abandon her during her illness. It was the first time in my life, someone close to me on a daily basis, was dying.

She was in the last stages of cancer and had been losing weight rapidly. Sandy came to my house with a new pair of slacks for me to hem because she had no energy for anything. As she slipped out of her dungarees, I gasped at the sight of her legs. She was a tall, thin girl to begin with, but now her legs were showing only bones, and the thigh skin drooped downward. I had to brace myself, after I became light-headed from seeing the reality of what happens physically to someone near death.

I was so frightened losing my friend and facing death head on, I ran from it. Instead of being there when she needed support and someone to talk to from depression, I'm ashamed to say, I left her facing it without me.

She lived two houses around the corner, and I stopped all visits. I acted on my own selfish fears. It was too close to me and I honestly didn't know how to handle it. Knowing she was leaving this world; frightened me beyond words.

Sandy was my age, in her early forties, and my thought was constantly, *What if the same thing happens to me?* If the situation was turned around, I've no doubt at all in my heart that she would've been by my bedside to help me take my last breath.

Her husband called at work informing me that Sandy was rushed to the hospital. Guilt overcame me and I finally decided to push my own fears aside, and to go to see her when I left for the day.

My time was not her time. Before leaving, I received a final call from a friend telling me Sandy had just passed away. My nerves completely unraveled, and I had to leave my cubicle in customer service to get myself back under control so I could finish the day. I started to comprehend, that time waits for no one. I should've separated my fears and realized, it was all about *her,* not me. Instead, I left her wondering how anything could be more important than our being friends.

We should've spent our last moments together laughing, asked for forgiveness if we hurt each other and talked about what we shared and enjoyed as friends. I had had a chance to give and show a friend love before she left this earth. I was too worried about how it affected me when she was the one dying and leaving. What an awful painful lesson I had to learn to live with.

Now I was trying not to repeat my selfish actions during my own father's illness. He had to feel the love from his family and the security of not being left alone when he needed us the most. It's all about the dying person…not us.

Chapter 7
Deciding Mom's Caregivers

In addition to the turmoil of Dad's sickness, my brother, Joe, and Marge, were trying to find a home with an in-law apartment. They wanted to take care of my parents so they could finally relax in their late years. Both of them still believed Dad was going to live. Leona worked part-time for a real estate business and helped them with the search.

Dad had already decided who would be the best person to leave Mom with once he was gone. He knew Leona provided the necessary security for my mother. She had given up high school in her senior year during Mom's breakdown to take care of her.

The breakdown caused my mother to have no memory of her life for six months. Close friends came to the house to help whenever they had free time. Leona stayed home so our father could continue going to work without being worried about leaving Mom alone.

My mother probably had postpartum after having my brothers so late in life. The doctors wanted to give my mother shock treatments and my father absolutely refused to put her through something so horrifying to him. Today there are all kinds of medicine and counseling to help women. Back then doctors didn't know what baby blues were that women suffered through.

February 10, 1955, Joe was born when Bill was four years old. Mom had had the boys in her middle forties with a fourteen year gap between me and Joe. The family thought that might have helped contribute to her breakdown. She couldn't handle the responsibility during that time of her life. Leona jumped right in with no regrets. My sister became a mother to the boys instead of a sister. She gave up her teen years with little time for her own friends. Not once did she ever complain, even to this day.

Dad must've had a hard time not choosing Leona to leave Mom with because she had spent the most years tending to her. Leona was now fifty-four years old, and the oldest. He came to the conclusion that her age was against her. My mother could live to be in her nineties like her mother. In twenty some years, Leona's health could fade and stop her from completing the responsibilities that Mom would need.

Albert was forty-nine years old and his sons, David and Dan, were in their twenties and still lived at home. Albert and Maria had their businesses to run.

I was next in line, also forty-nine, but my life was not stable enough being single. Debbie and Lori were both married with two children of their own. At the time, Al and I had no plans for marriage. I wouldn't be able to care for her being at a job every day.

Bill was thirty-nine years old and he and Sharon were expecting their first child in November. The catering business Sharon worked for often called for her to travel. Bill rode an hour to work and that would leave Mom alone. Bill and I both lacked the full time to become caregivers for Mom.

Joe and Marge were the two most reasonable choices in our father's opinion. They had no children and Joe was the youngest, at thirty-five-years old. Dad had the comfort and belief in his heart that Joe would be healthy and young enough to see Mom through her remaining years.

The perfect house was found in South Dennis. Because of his cancer, Dad didn't even try to bargain with the owners. He paid the asking price just to get the papers signed. My parent's home in East Falmouth was put on the market and it took a full year for it to sell.

The Cape home fit everything and everyone. It had three bedrooms, two full baths, a good sized living room and a full kitchen with sliding doors going out to a deck that wrapped around the kitchen. There was a full sized apartment with two bedrooms over the two-car garage where Joe and Marge would stay. Their upholstery business would be run out of the double door garage. We were all excited about the home and convenient location.

Chapter 8
Dad's Confession

Dad started to feel worse during his chemo treatments. Leona wanted to take him to the LaSalette Shrine in Attleboro. The location offers Mass, healing services, and confession. It's located in Southeastern Massachusetts and run by the priests. For over thirty years the Center has been a vital contributor to spiritual renewal for those seeking a deeper relationship with God.

My father hesitated at first, because he said something bothered him. As time passed, he finally decided to make the trip with her, along with Mom, Joe and Marge.

When they drove into the parking lot, Dad said, "I can't do this."

Leona replied back, "You don't have to get out of the car; just sit and feel the peace."

My father finally admitted he had not been to Confession for over thirty years. The statement shocked everyone because he had been a lecturer at Mass every week. He was a very active and devoted Catholic.

He feared death because he had fought and killed soldiers during WWII. Since the war, he was tortured mentally, thinking God would not forgive him and send him to Hell to suffer because of it.

Leona went into the main office and asked if a priest could hear his confession. The administrator called up to the Retreat House to see if a priest was available. She was told to bring Dad through another entrance and to not say a word to anyone where they were going. Confessions were not scheduled yet, and the priest didn't want to call attention to this special request before regular hours.

Dad spent twenty minutes with the priest in Reconciliation. When he walked out, Leona said the relief in his facial expression was plainly visible. No one asked what was said to him but they could see the peace of mind he had received.

He requested to walk on a path at the top of the hill behind the Stations of the Cross. It's a devotion consisting of prayers and meditations before each of the fourteen crosses or images set up along the church path commemorating the events of the Passion of Jesus.

To get there, they all had walked passed the forty, or so steps, that lead up to the crucifixion statue. From there, they traveled up a side path to reach the top. Hundreds of pilgrims have climbed them on their knees as penance. This time, my father wouldn't be one of them. There was no physical strength left in his body. The family helped him gently make his private pilgrimage to God. I know our Heavenly Father was aware of Dad's painful sacrifice and sincere piety at this time.

In 1985, my brother, Albert, had brought a video tape to East Falmouth for the family to watch. The event had been about six visionaries, ranging from ten to sixteen years of age, in a little town called Medjugorje in Bosnia. They were claiming to see and speak to Our Blessed Mother with the apparitions occurring every single day since June 24, 1981. Each visionary was receiving ten secrets from her that would be given to the world and change it forever. When the last one received all ten, the events would start unfolding.

Dad had been captivated as he watched the video. He mentioned how he would like to travel to Bosnia to witness the apparitions. I had the same fascination, but feared flying. Leona had never flown before, and swore never to travel by air.

Every so often, Dad would discuss the trip, but no one offered to go with him. It didn't take long for the subject to disappear.

It was now 1990, as Dad tried to make the LaSalette pilgrimage. Leona had remembered back that Dad wanted to go to Medjugorje.

She asked, "Dad, do you want me to take you to Medjugorje?"

"I'm too weak for that now, Leona," he said.

Leona's heart had filled with sadness knowing that she waited too long to ask the question. It was an effort for Dad to just get back to the car.

Chapter 9
Chemo Treatments Not Working

After seven months of chemo treatment, the doctor called my father, sadly stating, "I'm sorry, Al, but the treatment is not working. You need to get your things in order."

My father asked the horrifying question, "How long?"

"Two to four weeks."

Dad refused to believe what he just heard and Mom was panic stricken at the thought. All their years together were coming to an end.

My sister called me with the news and it felt like someone kicked me in my stomach. I was fighting fear and disbelief at the same time. My mind did not want to absorb any of this since I was still praying for a miracle.

After getting the news, I rushed to visit my parents the next night. When I entered the front door, they were sitting together on the couch in the living room watching television. I tried to brace myself with the sight of my father. My legs felt like jelly seeing Dad's trousers just hanging off him. They looked two sizes too big. Because they were so baggy, it allowed the complete outline of bones in his legs to show. My mind raced back to Sandy with the same thinness I had witnessed a few years earlier.

I couldn't believe how in the few short weeks, since my last trip to the Cape, Dad's condition worsened. I took a deep breath to compose myself before giving him a hug and kiss. Inside I was screaming with anger and panic for my parents and, selfishly, for myself. I was very aware this time, however, that this was not about me.

Mom asked if I wanted to have some hot chocolate and I accepted feeling she wanted time alone with me in the kitchen. I followed behind her and sat at the table. She went about collecting the ingredients and the pan needed to prepare the mix. It was always special because it was homemade. Before she added the milk to the chocolate that was already bubbling, the steam had filled the surrounding rooms with the delicious aroma. A strong whiff went through me and it brought back memories.

My thoughts traveled to when we were children and every winter, Mom would always have hot cocoa waiting for us after our sledding or ice skating events. Albert and I would prance into the house with all our friends. Nothing was more enticing than to see and smell the hot steaming cups of hot cocoa placed on the table. No matter how many friends were with us, Mom never voiced any complaint about there not being enough to go around. After coming into the entryway wet and cold with frozen snow on us, we would start stripping the layers of clothing off with incredible speed to get to the kitchen table.

Discovering marshmallows floating and melting on top only added to the treat. Some would pick it up slowly with their spoons so it would not burn their tongues. The rest of us would blow on it and then take short sips only to come up with a marshmallow mustache. My mother watched us many times, getting satisfaction from her loving action.

I came back to reality as Mom was pouring my hot chocolate. I knew this time it was a big project. She was not carrying the same satisfied look in her eyes as when we were younger. I could see her confused state as she tried to do a simple thing. Her heart was not in it. The months of stress and unanswered prayers had just drained her.

She sat down across from me at the kitchen table. Dad refused a cup, as he had done with everything else that was offered to him in the last few weeks. When he had a slight hunger for certain meals, Mom would immediately cook it, only to see him lose his appetite completely when she served it to him.

I asked Mom how she was doing because I was so wrapped up with Dad it was as if I had pushed her into the background. She had so much to deal with emotionally and physically within herself. All of us had our partners to go home to but my mother was trying to accept a future without a husband. I knew no matter how much she loved her children; we couldn't possibly fill his place.

He was no longer going to be there to hold her when she got lonely or comfort her when she got sick. Through the years, whenever Dad sat on the couch with Mom, he would always be seen rubbing his hand gently and slowly over her neck, shoulders or thigh without speaking a word. The same loving gestures he did for me when I was young. A touch is such a healing and comforting process and it is taken for granted, until the threat of its being gone forever is a reality. Being left at an old age, and facing life without your companion, had to be terrifying.

Mom looked at me after I asked the question and didn't know how to answer me. She was lost for words, as if her feelings were locked at the very bottom of her. She said Dad was very angry at the doctor. He refused to believe he was dying.

I asked if she wanted me to get in touch with Hospice to help the both of them. I thought if Hospice was there for her during this hard time, they may be there to give her the added support after his death. The organization could be the answer to give Mom the counseling that she has needed for years.

"Before I make a decision, I have to speak to your father. He has to approve of it first," she said.

I watched as she finally started to take short sips on her hot chocolate that had sat on the table for at least ten minutes. It must've turned cold while she had been talking, because the steam left the cup and she showed no desire to finish it.

My mother, Sophie Gramm, was seventy-six years old with absolutely no gray hair. She never looked her age and it always amazed us and her friends. Her sister, Helen, told me that when my mother was single, she was a stunning woman and had men flocking to her.

Mom spent hours in her yard. She enjoyed caring for the flowers and vegetable garden. She watered them every day: whether it rained or not. My mother had a green thumb, and everyone remarked how beautiful and healthy her flowers looked. I tried desperately to have the same striking flowers in my backyard. It failed, since I never kept up with the watering.

I worried about my mother, because my father had done everything for her. Dad had offered to teach her how to drive, but she never took advantage of the opportunity. The only way she would travel outside the house, was if a family member was with her. Since her breakdown, she feared doing anything alone.

Mom never got professional help to learn how to get her confidence and independence back. She feared doing anything on her own. I felt so bad and didn't know how to comfort her. I cleared off the table and cleaned the kitchen before leaving. Mom said she would let me know what Dad thought of the Hospice services as soon as she spoke to him.

The next night Leona called me screaming uncontrollably because she received a call from Dad and he was all upset. Mom had spoken to him about Hospice and he snapped at her, "Hospice! Why do I need them? They're for the dying and I'm *not* dying!"

My sister's investigation came to the conclusion that I was the one who planted the Hospice seed. Leona cried, "It took us months to convince Dad he was not going to die and now the family has to start giving him hope all over again because of what you did."

At the time, my concern was for my mother, and I had felt she and all of us needed the support from Hospice. I finally came to accept the reality that my father was dying, but found no peace with it. I believed in miracles, but at eighty years old, God had to be calling him. No one else in the family had given up hope. Joe was already in the process of trying to find a store with natural herbs to heal him. Meanwhile, Mom was walking around in a daze. She must have been in a state of panic knowing Dad was not going to be in her life.

I was stunned, that everyone in the family had not accepted the prognosis from the doctor. I seemed to be the only one facing Dad's outcome. He had everything against him: his age, cancer in his liver, stomach, and prostate. I felt like an enemy within the family unit from not holding onto hope.

Chapter 10
Getting Ready for the Move

Papers were finally signed for the house in South Dennis, and since there were no problems, my parents wanted to move in right away on Columbus Day weekend. Boxes were now being collected by everyone so we could start packing their belongings.

The next two weekends my girlfriend, Roberta Crealese, who worked with me, helped me get organized. She is in her early thirties with curly red hair and blessed with a firm body from her faithful and daily gym workouts. She's an energetic person who enjoys being active and boredom is not a part of her life.

Roberta was a tremendous help and moved like a pro, stuffing items into the right-sized boxes. I was very impressed with her speed in getting rooms cleaned out. From numerous moves in her single life, she had it down pat.

I moved in slow motion, accomplishing nothing. Everything I packed away only brought me to tears. Each article in my hand took me back to a period in my life with warm memories. I couldn't keep up with Roberta, who was doing ninety percent of the work. All I wanted to do was sit in a corner and pray for the black cloud that had engulfed our family to pass over us.

I knew deep down that Dad was fading when he lost his appetite and strength. These signs confirmed in my heart that his death was now a reality. Emotionally, I didn't want to let go. I couldn't foresee life without my father or the fact my mother was going to be left alone. Our family's solid foundation was falling apart. A move should be the beginning of hope and happiness, but this was not the case for Mom's future or ours.

The weekend for the move was upon us. Friday night, Al and I went to stay overnight to help my parents with the last minute details. Leona and my mother were in the living room watching television together when we entered the house. Albert was with Dad in his bedroom watching a Patriots football game. We decided to watch the game with them. As we cheered with each good play, I noticed how Dad loved having everyone around him. The loud excitement in the room seemed to put some life back in him.

The game ended and everyone moved back into the living room, leaving Dad alone. I stayed behind with my father and asked how he was doing.

Looking washed-out, he answered, "Not good at all. I've lost my strength to walk, and my freedom to get up and go anywhere."

Dad was worried and uncomfortable from not having had a bowel movement in five days. This was the first time he had ever spoken to me about any private issues. I tried not to make him uneasy talking about it.

I gave a few private suggestions on what he might do to help relieve the problem. I don't know how he had the strength to get off the bed and walk into the bathroom. My eyes filled up and a lump formed in my throat, seeing him so frail and weak as he walked in and closed the door.

After ten minutes, he came back into the bedroom and I could see his frustration. He looked at me and explained how painful it was when he tried.

I left him for a moment to go into the living room and mentioned to my mother what was happening. She was not concerned and said the doctor gave him pills for it and they would work sooner or later.

I looked at her and replied, "It has been almost a week! He must have an impaction. If he does, the pills won't help him."

I returned to Dad's bedroom and found him on the bed, completely exhausted from numerous times of trying after I had left him. He must've had terrible stomach pains. He was not eating much but that wouldn't prevent a blockage. I couldn't bring myself to walk out and leave him alone in this condition.

I saw Mom go into the other bedroom across the hall. After a good ten minutes or so, the realization came over me she was settling there for the night. I found an excuse to leave my father and went to see her. There she was under the covers with no intention of going anywhere else. I asked if she was going to join Dad.

Her reply was, "I haven't slept with your father for quite a while now."

I stood there paralyzed in shock wondering how she could've left him every night alone in his room. Mixed feelings of anger and pity for her ran through me. My imagination went wild thinking about how many days, weeks or months he had been left to think about his life ending and suffering with his pain. *How long has she been doing this to him?* I looked at her, questioning if there was a heart beating in her.

"Mom, I'm afraid he might fall out of bed," I said searching for any excuse to get her to go sleep with him.

She replied back in an angry and demanding voice, "Go to bed and stop worrying about him. He'll be fine."

My mind couldn't accept her coldness. She always used a certain tone to intimidate us so we would back off and leave her alone. This was one of those times.

She was trying not to face the situation and it protected her from the fact it was happening. At the moment, I didn't feel sorry for her because my thoughts were on my father who was sleeping alone. *My God! How can anyone be expected to sleep with their own death imminent?*

I returned to Dad and could see the panicked look in his eyes, and sensed from his body language from tossing and turning, that he feared being left alone. *Alone*...to think of your life slipping away from you, leaving your family, not to feel another human body next to you to receive comfort and security, not to have someone to talk to so your mind will not think about the death process. *Alone*...giving you time to imagine your body returning to the earth, wondering if God will find you worthy to be with Him in eternity, fearing of suffering in Purgatory.

All of these thoughts might have been running through his mind in the dark. *Alone!*

Approaching him, I saw a father who was once proud of his accomplishments in life. So many times our family was uprooted so he could accept higher positions in companies. This allowed him to give us more in life. Hard choices, like the ones he had to make as a commander for the servicemen under him during WWII. This heartless, vicious disease was slowly destroying him, leaving no way to fight back.

I went over and asked, "Dad, do you want me to lie with you a while on the other side of the bed?"

His eyes looked like the weight of the world had come off his shoulders. Being relieved he said, "Yes, I'd like that."

Peace seemed to flow over him when he realized he wasn't going to be alone. He had to be frightened to have his daughter stay with him.

Before settling down to rest beside him, I went into the bathroom. I was completely taken back discovering it hadn't been cleaned. *How could I have been so blind not to know my parents needed help? Where was my selfish heart all these months?* Mom was in no emotional state to worry about cleaning. Getting up and facing the day was her chore. *God forgive me.*

The end was here and there was no time to make up for what was not done for them. Without knowing it, I was doing the same thing of which I was accusing Mom. I hid at home to protect myself from seeing him fading away. The same thing I did with Sandy. What I was seeing and feeling in the five hours of being here couldn't possibly touch the heartbreak Mom was experiencing day in and day out all these months. It was almost midnight when I finished cleaning every inch of the bathroom, leaving it spotless.

Dad had turned off the lights and was resting in the darkness when I went back in the bedroom. I bent down to kiss him goodnight before settling at the corner of the bed. I placed my hand on top of his so he would feel the warmth of it and know he was not alone. This was my first real connection with my father. I stayed next to him until I could hear the last deep sigh from relaxing and knew he was in a deep sleep.

Chapter 11
Moving Day

Morning came and it was a beautiful warm, sunny day. There was no time to relax and sleep late because the movers were at the house early. Family members were running in different directions, finishing what had to be done to make the move go smooth and fast. Roberta pulled into the driveway to help pitch in again.

Camilla and Dante Picciano were standing in the kitchen after coming through the path in the backyard to see Dad. This was not a normal visit from them and they knew this would be their final farewell. None of this was going to be easy.

After greeting them, I went to get my father. I rounded the corner and couldn't see him in the bedroom. When I stepped in a little further, I saw him in the bathroom. There he was, sitting on the closed toilet lid with only his trousers and a white t-shirt on. He was stretched over the sink, trying to shave. The left side of his face was resting on the side of the sink. He was struggling to shave with the razor in his right hand.

My heart sank in my chest. Never had I seen such a heartbreaking sight. He was determined to do it without bothering anyone again. I came up to him and asked if I could help. He handed me the razor and I tried carefully not to hurt him doing such a task. As the blade was brought down slowly, I watched not to cut his cheekbones. It was not a thorough job because his face was so thin that I couldn't get the razor around his jaw line.

Once I had helped Dad wash, I put him into the cushioned seat of a wheelchair that was provided for him from the hospital. When we entered the kitchen, the Piccianos were no longer waiting. Someone told me Mom informed them my father was not up yet. I walked through the path to their backyard and they were nowhere to be found. Later I learned they left to do some shopping, thinking we would be there on their return. The chance never came because we left before they came back.

Mom was still saying goodbye to the neighbors as I pushed the wheelchair out into the driveway. Cathi Valeriani, who was the vice president of the Ashumet Valley Property Owners, Inc., had arrived to see my father. Dad had been the secretary for the association for three years. Since Cathi lived only a block away, she and my father would meet often to work together. I could see the heartbreak in Cathi. Like so many coming to say goodbye, she knew this may be her last time to ever see him. I noticed Cathi's eyes fill up, and she struggled to keep herself in control.

After all the farewells, we put Dad in Leona's car. Everyone was choked-up as we watched him take a last look at his home before pulling away. It was the hardest thing in the world to hold back my tears in front of Al. I sat in our car and turned to face the window trying to hide my wet cheeks. My father had to be fighting the same emotions.

The cars that had lined up in the group had slowly started to pull away. I turned one more time to look at my parents' home. I imagined Dad at the end of the driveway waving his hand high in the air saying goodbye. Knowing he would never be seen doing this again made my heart break. It choked me up.

Roberta was right behind us, with her car packed full. South Dennis was thirty minutes away, and by the time we arrived, Dad was totally exhausted. It was my first time to see the new home. The movers had ninety percent of the furniture in place. It was a beautiful Cape Cod home in a nice neighborhood with plenty of woods around the sides and back of the house.

We took Dad around in the wheelchair to see all the rooms. At the end of the hall was my parent's bedroom. Two small windows filled their room with bright sunlight. Their canopy bed fit perfectly to the left of the entrance with the headboard centered against the wall. Their large dresser and mirror was on the opposite wall, facing the doorway, and gave the effect of the room appearing larger than it actually was.

I kept praying, "Please God, give Dad time to enjoy this place for awhile." He finally had come to live with Joe and Marge so they could help take so many burdens off his shoulders. Before Dad's cancer, Joe and my parents talked often about finding a home together. Now they were together for different reasons.

The full day of moving made everyone physically and mentally exhausted. We now had to face the heavy traffic leaving the Cape. We called it a night and headed back to our respective homes.

Chapter 12
Calling Hospice

The following Friday night I returned and stayed for the weekend. My first concern was finding out if the laxatives had helped my father. He informed me that he still hadn't had any relief from the problem. I talked with Joe and insisted Hospice should be called. He was uncomfortable with the idea knowing Dad was going to be upset. I was willing to take the complete blame. Leaving him in this condition was worse than him being angry at me.

Hospice informed Joe that they would only come if Dad's doctor ordered the service and if the patient agreed. Joe called the doctor and he was very much in favor of the organization coming to the house. The hardest thing was going to be to get our father to approve.

I went in his bedroom and explained Hospice would come to help him but he had to agree on their services. He skipped the statement and asked me if it would be painful to have a procedure for an impaction done. I told him that was something only a medical person could answer but I stressed to him that he couldn't stay like this. It was unhealthy and it could poison his system.

To my amazement, he agreed. I had no idea what had changed his mind but was not about to question it. It was 8:00 pm when Joe made the call to the doctor. He said he would make the arrangements with Hospice and they would send someone right away.

Within an hour, I answered the doorbell. Standing in the doorway was a girl from the Hospice Association of Cape Cod, Inc. from Yarmouthport. Little did we know the stress this organization was going to take off all our shoulders.

She smiled brightly and said, "Hi, I'm Cathy."

She was so tiny that the tote bag she was carrying in her hand seemed bigger than her. Cathy surprised me with her casual dress of sweats and sneakers. She seemed like the girl next door and her demeanor was very down to earth. She came through the front door carrying a handful of Hospice pamphlets. I introduced myself and led Cathy down the narrow hallway to Dad's bedroom. He smiled warmly to welcome her as she entered. Cathy's glance back in my direction told me they needed time alone.

I turned and joined the rest of the family in the kitchen. Joe, Albert, Bill and Leona were at the table with Mom. We all grouped together in conversation feeling a little tension with the reality of someone from Hospice in our home.

It was not long before Cathy came directly to the table and started to discuss Dad's condition. When she bent down to open her tote bag, I realized she was pregnant. She was wearing a large sweatshirt, and I hadn't noticed her condition.

She placed the pamphlets down on the table in front of us and suggested we read them when we had time. She emphasized that if there were any questions or problems, she was on call twenty-four hours, seven days a week. It wouldn't take her long to get here since she lived only ten minutes away.

Cathy then proceeded to tell the family, step by step, what to expect as Dad's health declined. She explained the availability of services and detailed how their volunteers could stay with him. The free time would allow the family to shop or just take a break from the stress. The volunteers also would clean the house and bathe Dad.

We listened with no comments and asked very few questions. It felt like we were passing through a bad nightmare. Cathy knew from her experience not to throw too much at us, or to overstay her first visit. She was wise to the fact that families had difficulty trying to deal with the last stages of a loved one's life.

I went in to see Dad after Cathy left. He looked relieved, but remarked on how painful and uncomfortable the procedure had been for him. I tried to assure him he would now start feeling much better. Going home Sunday would be easier for me, knowing he was no longer suffering from a blockage.

The following Monday night I received a call from him. He was yelling at me, claiming I didn't tell him the nurse that had come to see him was from Hospice. My father wanted nothing to do with the service anymore.

He was angry. "I'm not going to die and Hospice is for the dying. Why would you call them?"

I explained he must have misunderstood because I was honest about where Cathy was from. *Please God give me the right words to say to him.* I didn't know what was going to give him comfort about keeping the service. I only knew deep down all of us needed Hospice.

Finally, I said, "Dad, God decides who is going to die and when. Just because Hospice is there helping you does not mean the decision comes from them. If He wants you to live, you will."

I continued by saying, "You always worried about Mom being alone." Leona had told me that he had broke down crying in East Falmouth, staying he felt guilty leaving Mom alone. He was deeply aware how she depended on him, and she was horrified being left behind.

I tried to use this statement to help him decide to keep the service, if for no one else, but her. I continued, "If something does happen to you, Hospice will be there to help her cope. You make the decision, Dad. I was only trying to help the both of you. If you don't want Hospice, I will stand behind you."

A long silence came when he hesitated and then answered, "It'll be all right. They can continue to come."

God put the words in my mouth because my mind was blank for answers, since I hadn't been prepared for the call.

Chapter 13
My Brother Walter

A new girl arrived from Hospice introducing herself as Debbie. She was going to be the private nurse who would be handling all of Dad's medical problems. She started by telling the family to never use the word *pain* with any description to a patient. We were to say *discomfort*. "Pain," she expressed, "brings their mind directly to the cancer."

Debbie decided it was time to start him on morphine. She chose me to administer the medicine and my heart was in my throat with the idea. It was to be placed under his tongue. I looked at it as medicine that would keep him sedated all the time.

Debbie assured me the dropper contained only 5 mg and it was the lowest strength at least to start. This amount would only take the edge off the pain and still allow him to be aware of things happening around him. He would then be more comfortable and could communicate with us more easily.

I was so absorbed with Dad that I didn't want to leave his side. I can't remember if I took time to talk to my mother. Sharon and Maria, my sister-in-laws, were now staying over every weekend and spent most of the time with Mom. We placed two rocking chairs in his room, facing him. I chose the large one because it was his favorite rocker to sit in when he smoked his pipe.

Bill and Sharon were expecting their first child in November and the time was close. Emotions were high praying for Dad to hold out one more month to see the baby. He truly believed it would be a boy and talked about the things Bill could do with him. Albert's boys, David and Dan, were the only ones who would carry on the Gramm name.

It was extremely rare that my brother, Walter's, name was ever brought up in any family conversations. My parents had a difficult time talking about him.

My mother told me stories about him more freely before I became a teenager. She talked about the time she took Leona, Walter, Albert and me to a park. I'm not even sure where it was at the time. A man approached her, explaining he was a photographer and wanted to take pictures of us. Dad was stationed away from home at the time and she wanted his opinion on taking us. My father thought it was safe since he wanted her to go to his studio. She dressed the four of us up in our best clothes.

Mom said he focused a lot on Walter and did something very unusual. When the pictures were printed, there was one photo drawing of Walter done in pencil. He drew Walter with angel wings. No one knew, then or now, why this man saw Walter this way. I heard about this picture so many times but never saw it.

Another odd occurrence happened when Mom was ironing one day and Walter came up to her and asked, "Mommy, is it all right to love God more than your parents?"

She was completely taken back by the question and replied, "Yes, you *are* supposed to love God more than anyone else."

After he got his answer, he ran off to play but it left her trying to understand why this strange question, out of nowhere, was asked, sending chills through her.

It was not long after that when Walter got sick with polio and passed away. Boston had an epidemic of the disease and the hospitals ran out of iron lung machines. He was not fortunate to obtained one to help him breathe.

When Dad's illness got bad, he put the picture of Walter out in the open. He placed it on his bureau first in Falmouth, and then in South Dennis. The picture was in view for everyone to see, next to him. It was a piece of artwork left with many questions and no answers. A stranger saw Walter with wings. Why? Did he know something?

My mother had a breakdown and carried guilty feelings about Walter's death for years. She told me about the bus trip coming home after spending a full day shopping in the city with Walter, Leona, Albert and myself. Handling twins alone must have been a handful, let alone two other children.

Walter was being a normal brother, teasing the rest of us. It couldn't have been easy pulling four kids from store to store, and then fighting for seats on a bus while carrying heavy bundles. Mom was completely without patience from exhaustion.

She got aggravated with him and said, "I'll *never* take you to the city again!"

The chance never came before he died. The statement ate at her for years. She grieved for over twenty years until she had a spiritual experience. Dad had confirmed that he had witnessed the event. When Mom was in bed, her face suddenly lit up like a flashlight was under her skin.

My mother heard God say, "Let Walter go so he can come to Me. Your tears are holding him back."

Dad took her to a priest the next day to confirm her vision. She was completely at peace after this. My mother was told by Our Heavenly Father that Walter had been in a floating state waiting to go to Heaven since he was seven. She wasn't sure if He meant Purgatory. Mom was holding him from eternal peace with her own personal pain.

I was intrigued learning she had heard God's voice. I wanted more than anything to feel what that blessing was like. I questioned her so many times wanting a description of what His voice sounded like. My mother tried explaining there are no words on this earth to describe it except that His voice was so peaceful.

Dad went through the same guilty feelings with Walter's death. One day as he and I sat in the den in East Falmouth, he shared his own story with me. He had also taken the four of us to a park in Worcester and was very upset with Walter.

Walter had been fussy all day and Dad said to him, "I'll *never* take you to the park again."

I sat there watching the tears pouring down my father's cheeks with his head down in his hands, crying uncontrollably.

He looked up at me absolutely heartbroken. "It has been over forty years and I still can't forgive myself for saying that to him. I never had the chance to take him again!"

It was the first time in my life I saw my father cry. It was a hidden side of him. He never before showed any emotions in front of me. I can't remember to this day what I said to comfort him. My memory of that moment was only seeing his innermost feelings from losing a child. They both took his death very hard.

Mom had mourned and wept for years before this apparition with God. She couldn't bring herself to go to Walter's grave site in Worcester. The visitation from God had helped her to know her tears and pain kept him from entering Heaven. Mom and Dad had to let go and trust in Our Lord to take care him. After all, he was back home. My parents are now at peace. Crying innocently holds souls from moving toward God. It's a lesson I never forgot.

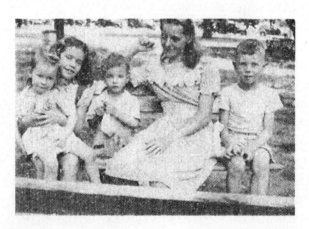

Left Front: Alberta, Leona, Albert, Mom & Walter

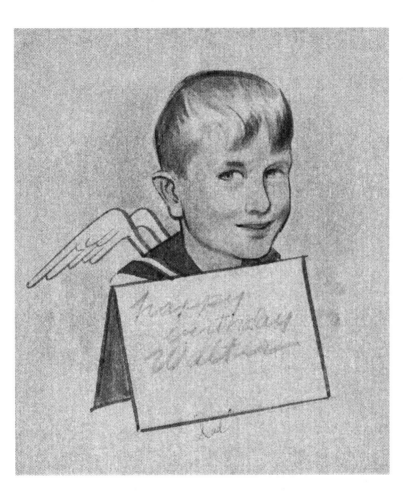

Walter with Angel Wings

Chapter 14
Friends Saying Farewell

Dad was tremendously weak and slept most of the day. My parent's military friends were all notified of the short length of time we had left with him. The couples started to come each day to say their final farewell.

A former General in his eighties, who served with Dad during WWII, came to visit him. I peeked through the bedroom door that was cracked open slightly to make sure he was awake and alert enough to respond to his visitor. There the man sat in Dad's big rocker with his back towards me. He was leaning over, talking very closely to my father in bed and reminiscing about their times together in the service.

I could see Dad blinking his heavy eyelids. He was continuously trying to fight to keep them open. He wanted to show interest in what the General was saying to him. Between his weakness and the effect of the morphine, he was in and out during the whole conversation.

I couldn't understand how the gentleman was not aware of Dad's eyes being closed as he spoke to him. Maybe there was something that had to be said between friends before his passing.

Out of all the dearest and truest friends, one special couple didn't show to see him. Joe and Anita St. Onge were so close to the whole family that, as kids and right through to our adulthood, we called them Uncle Joe and Aunt Anita.

Joe had met my father when they both worked at the American Bosch Company in Springfield. He joined the National Guard at the same time as Dad but served in a different infantry during WWII. After the service, wherever my father worked, Joe followed him to the same company. My father retired as President of Pyrotector, Inc. in Hingham, and Joe stayed there until his own retirement, ten years later.

Joe and Dad had a problem between them that they couldn't resolve. The two couples had to deal with a situation that separated them for over twenty years. Dad never talked about Joe without getting choked up and it was even worse during his illness. My father told me he never had a more devoted friend and was completely lost all the years without him. My father was an only child and Joe became an inseparable brother to him. They did everything together. With his days declining, Dad spoke to me again about Joe. I could sense the mental strain and frustration he was under from wanting to repair the friendship before he died. It was so obvious that the love in his heart for Joe was tearing him apart inside. He wasn't in a position to make the call, so I prayed for God to give me the strength to get involved and do what had to be done.

Joe lived about four miles from my home in Dighton. I had never stopped visiting him or my aunt because of the conflict. I made the call and told him the end was near and how my father longed to see him. I informed him exactly how Dad felt about the loss of their friendship over the years.

I begged him to bury the disagreement so they could both say what was in their hearts before it was too late. I couldn't live with myself, knowing my father died without asking for or receiving forgiveness. I promised to be there when he came. Joe asked me to give him a few days to prepare himself. He told me that my father was such a strong man and leader that he couldn't handle seeing him so frail and defeated. He was doing the same thing I'd done to Sandy.

Four days later, Joe arrived, unannounced. He walked through the kitchen door, joking and hugging as he always did. I knew his teasing and wit were a cover-up to hide how awkward he must have felt in this situation. He was very uncomfortable facing my mother after all the years of not keeping in touch. This had to be the hardest thing in the world for Joe to do. He didn't know how to face my father after the foolish years that were wasted not seeing each other and now had to confront the reality that his best friend was dying.

Dad had no idea Joe entered the house until he came around the corner into the living room. My father was sitting in the wheelchair in front of the bay window soaking up the sun in a daze, as if he was day dreaming. I don't think Joe got completely through the doorway when he broke down. He got on his knees at the foot of the wheelchair and embraced my father. They both held onto each other and sobbed.

The pain hit me hard, knowing two friends had wasted so many years because of false pride. One would have to be blind not to see the love between them. I turned around and left them alone to say their goodbyes. Dad was never told I made that call to Joe. My father was left with the feeling he came from his own free will. That visit had to be one of the greatest gifts for my father.

Chapter 15
Reactions to the Cancer

I had been visiting my parents for a week, but it seemed like a month. Finding humor during Dad's illness was really hard. One day it came without us even looking for it. Our father often asked to have his head rubbed because it somehow brought him comfort.

One afternoon, Leona was fulfilling his request as she rested on his bed next to him. I was returning to the bedroom and stopped at the doorway. The mirror to the bureau was facing me and it reflected Leona and Dad on the bed together, sleeping. Leona's hand was still in a cup-like position on the top of his head after having massaged it.

To add to the scene, she was snoring loudly with her mouth wide open from exhaustion. Not expecting to see this, it immediately struck my funny bone to the point that I couldn't stop laughing at the sight. I went to get the others to share the moment to brighten the day. We all stood at the doorway, which made it all the more hilarious. Our roars did not wake either of them.

Each night came and went and Mom was still not sleeping with Dad in the new house. I mentioned this action to Cathy when she arrived the next day, because all of us found it cruel for her to not comfort him in this way.

Cathy explained this was a very normal reaction from a person being left behind, especially with the elderly. She said Mom was actually mad at him for making her face the time left on earth alone and she was scared.

"Your mother is running from the situation and is trying not to deal with it. Try to be patient and she'll come to terms with it in her own time," she replied.

I started to be more understanding of Mom's actions after Cathy told me this. I was so caught up in my own emotions that I by passed her feelings. She was probably very aware of what she was doing but did not know how to comfort Dad without falling apart herself. I passed this information along to the other family members so they wouldn't continue to hold her actions against her.

Cathy was concerned because I was not leaving Dad's bedside. I tried explaining how important it was that I embrace every moment left with him. As foolish as this may sound, I was afraid that after his death time would make me forget what he looked like. I wanted to have my father's face embedded into my mind forever. She insisted I cut the time I spent with him down, instead of being there all day long.

Cathy told the family this was now the time to begin allowing only two people at a time in his bedroom. She explained, "You have to understand, the dying don't want to let go if they hear everyone around them. It's a gift to them if you let *them* decide when to leave you. It would be nice to make a comfortable atmosphere for him with soft music. It'll keep your dad at peace with no confusion going on around him. You'll get a sign he is getting ready to leave when he starts leaving his belongings with family members."

Joe and Marge went immediately to their apartment and retrieved their stereo system when Cathy left the house. In minutes it was set-up in Dad's bedroom and we were trying to decide on what music to play for him. Christmas was not far off and Joe decided on Christmas music.

The first song he chose was *Silent Night* and my throat felt like it was going to bust from the throbbing pain holding back tears. I didn't want to face the truth that he was not going to be with us these up-coming holidays. *How are we all going to handle Thanksgiving and Christmas?* To this day, the sound of Christmas music, and especially that song, brings an overwhelming sadness and emptiness in my heart.

I have to walk away from people, whether I'm at home or in a mall, to be alone to compose myself. And at the same time, the pain brings him back to me. *Oh God! Please stop this from happening. Make it all go away.*

I noticed how seldom it was that Mom was in Dad's room. Days would go by without her going in at all. She was constantly cooking to make healthy meals so we would all keep our strength up. It kept her busy and out of Dad's room helping to avoid the sight of her husband slowly passing away. I honestly do not remember leaving his room to eat. It's erased from my mind. I couldn't cut down, or stay out of my father's room, after Cathy had asked me.

Chapter 16
Taking Two Weeks out of Work

It was the second Sunday night that I was leaving my parents to go home for the week. I would be returning the following Friday night to repeat the routine. I went into Dad's bedroom to say goodbye only to discover him in a deep sleep. I looked down at him and studied his face when a rush of fear came over me from nowhere. *If I leave tonight, I'll not see him alive next Friday,* I thought.

The feeling was so deep and overpowering inside me that I felt like someone was trying to warn me. It was so real that I went into the den and paced back and forth like a lion in a cage from the state of panic. For the first time, I was losing control and my nerves were coming apart.

Marge came in and saw me in this condition. "Alberta, what is the matter? What happened?"

I started to hyperventilate, "If I leave tonight, I'll not see my father alive again."

She got very upset. "What are you talking about? He's going to live. I don't want to hear this!" She and Joe were still holding onto a miracle.

I calmly and lovingly looked straight at her, "Marge, Dad's dying! He is eighty years old with cancer all through him. You have to accept this."

She left the room in tears, refusing to listen to me.

I stayed the night and the following morning I called my boss,

Trisha, at Perkins Paper. I told her I wouldn't be returning to work for two weeks. She was shocked and thought she did not hear me clearly.

She repeated back to me, "You're telling me, Monday morning, with this short notice, that starting *today* you're not coming in for two weeks?"

I didn't care at that moment if my position with the company was gone. The need to be with my parents was too strong. I knew that family was more important than a job. People are the ones who can't be replaced…a job could be. I wanted to be there to the end with him. I had no doubt whatsoever that these inner feelings were given to me from above.

I hung up, hoping she would understand, and felt guilty at the same time. It was the kind of position that if one person didn't show-up, the others had to take the overload and it doubled their stress.

I walked into Dad's bedroom and noticed how uncomfortable he seemed with the three pillows under him. They were causing his head to tilt forward and it left him in the most uncomfortable position. I decided to give him my soft pillow that went everywhere with me when I traveled. It was the only thing that helped relieve my own pain from an old neck injury caused from a car accident.

There was a selfish second of hesitation to take it to him because without it there was a chance of my waking up with excruciating, throbbing pain in both my neck and head. A hard pillow puts pressure on the nerves in my neck which also makes me nauseated for hours.

"You don't look comfortable and my pillow is very soft. Let's try it," I suggested.

He looked up at me, surprised, when I took one pillow away and added mine to the pile.

I tried picking the softest one in his pile to bring to my room as my replacement. Dad gave a sigh of relief when I lowered him onto the three pillows, with mine on top. To my amazement, I never suffered without my pillow after giving him mine. I believed that God gave me a gift, after I was willing to suffer my pain to give Dad comfort.

Chapter 17
Rosaries and Prayers

It was nighttime when I was sitting in my father's bedroom with Leona, Marge and Maria, as we watched Dad trying to pray the rosary. Even with his weakness, he was still devoted. When he fought in Europe during WWII, he promised God that if He brought him home safe to his family, he would say a rosary everyday until his death. That promise was never broken and he was struggling to keep it.

Leona leaned over and asked him, "Do you want us to say them and you can follow along with us?"

He looked up at her and said, "Yes, I'd like that," in a frail tone.

Marge and Leona disappeared to collect their personal rosaries. When Leona returned, she noticed that Maria and I had none in our hands. We both felt embarrassed and acknowledged not owning one and having absolutely no idea on how to say them. Leona searched around the house until she found two extras rosaries.

The Rosary is divided into five decades. Each decade represents a mystery or event in the life of Jesus and Mary. There are four sets of "Mysteries of the Rosary" *(Joyful, Luminous, Sorrowful, and Glorious)*.

Maria and I followed along as Marge and Leona took turns leading us through each mystery of the rosary. I was amazed they knew it by heart. Dad moved his fingers along each bead while his eyes were closed. I realized, for the first time, what the rosary was all about in prayer.

Not many children learn the rosary when they receive them for First Holy Communion. "The family that prays together: stays together!" How many times have we all heard that statement? I stopped my Catholic practice a good fifteen years ago. I had no desire to learn the rosary or go to church during the bad times in my marriage. I felt like God abandoned me with all my prayers.

When my marriage fell apart, my belief fell apart. I wanted to be a devoted wife and mother while I was fighting to hold my family together along with my sanity.

Sundays, when I was attending Mass, I took Debbie and Lori to church so God would be a part of their life until they left home and decided on what they wanted to practice. That's how I thought, until my world came falling down during one Mass.

As I stepped out of my pew to receive Communion, the line came to a halt. Out of nowhere, I started to feel smothered between the person in front and behind me. During this reaction, I tried not to become anxious by taking deep breaths and telling myself to calm down.

When the line started to move forward, my knees were shaking to the point where I feared my legs were not going to support me much longer. A hot sweat developed on my skin and I could only focus on what was happening. I didn't understand the reason for this physical condition taking over me.

My first thought was to get out of line but feared it would bring the parishioner's attention to me. I held onto the end of each pew with my right hand to keep from falling to the floor. *Please God, help me get to the altar and get through whatever is happening to me.* I'd never experienced this before, and was panicking.

Today Holy Communion is not served like it was back then. Eucharistic Ministers now help the priests keep the line moving at a steady and faster pace. I finally made it up to the priest to receive and couldn't get back to my seat fast enough. I was so out of control, my hands were trembling and my heart was pounding through my chest. I was fighting nausea and it was making me sick.

I grabbed my two girls and left before Mass ended. I felt only anger at God. *How could You do this to me? Here I'm trying to hold everyone together. Why are these terrible things happening to me?*

The stress at home was affecting my nerves but I didn't understand this at the time. My ex-husband and I fought often when he came home from drinking. He would be in blackouts and I tried to control his anger, so my children would be protected from hearing and witnessing the constant battles. The up and down emotions affected me mentally and physically. I couldn't handle going anywhere for months.

The fear of losing control in church again kept me away for years. After that incident, the same response happened when I went into any public place and was pushed into a crowd.

I suddenly lost my independence and confidence to go anywhere. If I could get in and out right away, or attend functions knowing I could get up and leave if I wanted, then I could handle it. Otherwise, I stayed within the safety of my home. It took a long time before I realized that my body had been pushed beyond what it could take physically and emotionally.

Now here I sat, with family, holding a rosary. Our purpose was to say it for Dad but I felt something happening inside me. I decided to offer it up as my gift for my father's soul.

I once read the book, *Life After Life*, by Raymond Moody, and it related personal stories about people in the process of dying and what they felt and saw during their passing over to the other side. They all remarked about being pulled toward a light and sensed if they went toward it, they would not return. The light was telling them about the need for prayers, forgiveness and love for each other on earth. Any article on death now fascinated me and I couldn't read enough about it.

I had a similar experience after reading Moody's book. Bob and Leona were invited to join Debbie, Lori and myself for dinner at our home in Dighton. I was eating corn when something funny was said at the table, and it started me laughing. I was walking to the kitchen from the dining room, when suddenly, a kernel of corn went down my throat the wrong way, and I couldn't breathe.

Bob jumped up and came running behind me with one hand across the other and started to push inward below my rib cage. There was no pain or fear at that moment. I never heard Debbie on the phone next to me calling for an ambulance.

I remember swiftly and abruptly going into myself and had a sense of being separated from my body. It felt like I was in complete darkness, without losing consciousness. I had the impression my eyes were looking out through cut holes in a solid, gloomy, wall into a lighted room. I had no feeling of my body at all.

I thought, *Soon I'll see a light and go into the other world.* I waited for it with excitement. There was complete peace without any fright, and I was in a state of total tranquility. At that very moment, I noticed Leona and Lori crying hysterically. My next thought was, *Oh, Lord, I don't want them to see me die in front of them.* At that instant, I came out of the darkness and saw everything normally. I was brought back to my surroundings, and was aware of Bob trying to help me.

It was a wonderful experience. I truly believe, it was the beginning of leaving this earth. My family said I was chocking—I only remember looking for the light.

Chapter 18
Dad Distributing His Memorabilia

Al came to my parents' home, telling me he'd made a deposit of five-hundred dollars into my checking account to help toward my bills. There were no words to show him my appreciation. He was a very giving person and took care of anything that had to be repaired or replaced at my home. I held three jobs to support my girls and the house. If there was anything he saw the three of us needed, he gave it. I was blessed with a special man in my life.

God bestowed me with more abundance. Roberta arrived and delivered a card from my co-workers. They collected over four-hundred dollars from the employees, salesmen and the managers. I had more money than if I'd gone to work. God was surely taking care of me.

Bill and Sharon started to stay over at our parent's house more often and Sharon helped Mom with the cooking. The whole family worried about her being pregnant and under so much stress.

The next day, my father called the boys into his bedroom and started to pass out some of his service collections. Dad gave Bill the German sword he confiscated during WWII. Albert received Dad's rifle, the one with which he had won three National Rifle Association Marksmanship titles during the 1930s. He tried to give Leona all his service medals because she took them out so often to look at and study, but she felt all his Army memorabilia should be left to his sons, so the medals were passed down to Joe. He was now doing what Cathy said would happen before letting go. I thought his time must be near the end.

The following night my father had difficulty breathing, so Cathy was called to come over to confirm he was all right. When she arrived, she went straight to his bedroom and closed the door to have a personal conversation with him. I wondered how she performed this emotional work while pregnant. She never showed any signs of being tired or over-burdened.

Cathy gave us peace of mind when she came out of the room, saying our father was fine for the moment. When she was ready to go, I walked her to the door. It was a beautiful, warm night and the clear sky was aglow with millions of stars. We decided to sit together on the front steps and just relax. She had given such support that I wanted her to know from my heart what she meant to the family.

I opened up to her and said, "Cathy, you and the girls from Hospice are angels from heaven. Without the service, we would've been doing everything all wrong."

It taught me that there is no need for any family to go through this heartbreak and stress alone when an organization like this one exists.

Each night we continued with the rosary, only to see Dad's concentration leaving him. He could no longer follow the beads with his fingers; he would try, then completely stop and close his eyes.

I had become aware of all the decades of the mysteries of the rosary. I learned what they meant and it allowed me to pray from my heart and feel that the closeness of God was all around me. I talked to Jesus not only through prayer, but in my thoughts during the daily tasks I did for Dad. I could feel God's presence and my strength was coming from a source other than myself. It is hard to explain: the strain was there, but so was the comfort.

We called the Holy Trinity Church in Harwich to request our father receive Holy Communion everyday. He had trouble swallowing and had completely stopped eating. One morning while Dad received, he started to choke. I asked the priest if Dad was unable to take the host anymore, perhaps I could take it for him.

Dad jumped right in and said, "No, I'll take it myself!" No matter how sick he was, he could handle taking the Eucharist.

With each visit, the priest placed his hand on Dad's shoulder gently and said, "Continue on your journey, Al." I was heartsick, knowing anytime he could be taken from us.

The next afternoon Marge and I massaged Dad's legs with body lotion when we noticed his feet felt cold. As I placed the blankets on top of him, I remarked, "Your feet are freezing, Dad. Let me warm them up for you."

He looked up shocked and smiled when he replied, "They don't feel cold to me."

I informed Cathy with her next visit about the small incident. She told us to stop massaging any body parts because it would only spread the cancer faster. The family talked it over and felt that nothing was going to stop his dying process. Since it gave him such pleasure, we decided to continue, without saying anything to Cathy. After all, what other human contact did he have?

Chapter 19
Our Last Weekend

Debbie arrived from Hospice the next morning and gave Dad his daily examination. She then came into the kitchen to talk to the family. Calmly and directly, she informed us this would most likely be our last weekend with our father. Her years and experience working with the terminally ill gave her the insight on what to expect and when death would occur.

Albert and Joe got up and left the table to go outside. Neither of them could handle the news; they didn't want to hear this from her. The rest of us sat there in denial with Mom. I felt my insides shaking and feared losing control of myself. On the outside, I looked completely composed but only God knew what was happening to me on the inside. As Debbie kept talking to us, I wanted to run out the door and scream as loudly as possible.

She tried to explain to us the medical signs of when a person is ready to pass away. "His kidneys are shutting down and I can tell this by the brown color in his urine. That is usually what happens at the end. The last thing the dying loses is his hearing, so he will be aware of things being said for awhile."

The words made me so sick to my stomach that I thought it was going to make me throw-up. *Oh, God, I thought I had a hold on this!* I knew—we all knew—it was coming, but actually hearing he would be gone by the end of the week, brought all the underlying fears and feelings to the surface. There was now a time limit placed on how long we had left with him.

I was struggling emotionally to keep in control in front of my mother, but I could feel myself unraveling. I felt dizzy and faint. I feared a breakdown was going to shatter me into pieces. How could one remark affect me so badly both physically and mentally? I tried to block out Debbie's voice in an effort to get a grip on my surroundings and myself.

I sensed everyone at the table felt the same way. Not one of us could give support to the other. When Debbie finished talking, she left and not one person spoke. We were all trying not to give way to our tears in front of our mother. Each person went their separate way to deal with their own emotions. Somehow, I got up from the table without breaking down and crying. I could feel it deep down and wanted to release it, but nothing surfaced.

I was frantic now to hold onto every last moment with my father. I sat in his rocking chair for hours, my eyes constantly fixed on him as he slept. This was going to be my last week with him. I didn't want to let go and couldn't imagine life without him in it.

As I rocked slowly, I watched him. He was in a deep sleep. There was no music playing, no other person in the bedroom. It was a time for us alone. My mind started to drift in prayer and I tried to speak to my father spiritually.

Dad, miracles happen, don't they? God, don't take him from me. He is the frame to our family. Prayers are answered, but deep down I knew his life was over and that God was calling him back. I looked at the drawing of Walter that sat on his tall bureau with the angel wings. *Is Walter waiting for you?* I wondered.

Without any warning, my father opened his eyes, gave me a warm, loving smile, and held direct eye contact with me for a few moments. It was the same soft smile he had given me throughout my life. His gaze penetrated my eyes and went right through to my heart. As always, the smile said so much without words. He showed such alertness that it was hard to believe he was even ill.

I smiled back, hoping my love reached him the same way. He closed his eyes, giving us no time to converse. Little did I know there would never be another time I would see him awake. His smile was the most powerful gift he could have given me. It was a shared time that would never leave me. It was as if he woke up long enough to say goodbye to me.

Chapter 20
Dad's Passing

Maria was leaving Sunday night to go back to work at the hair salon on Monday and Albert was going to continue the vigil with the family. She felt uncomfortable with the decision fearing she wouldn't see Dad alive again, and left crying about it. She would be returning the following Friday for the weekend. We said goodbye and I tried to assure her that he would be waiting. I felt uneasy telling her that because I had the same fear.

Tuesday night, Mom finally told us she was going to sleep next to Dad and that it was something she had to do. It must have been so difficult for her even though she had slept next to him for over fifty years.

By now, I'd lost ten pounds. Waking up during the middle of the night was a normal thing for all of us, and getting back to sleep was sometimes impossible. My body felt like it weighed a ton each morning. After only a few hours sleep, family members were connecting in the kitchen frequently during the night.

Friday morning, I woke up and heard the television playing softly in the living room. The clock revealed it was only four in the morning. Walking toward the sound half awake, I found Leona sitting on the couch, watching the early morning shows with the volume low.

She admitted to not being able to sleep. It was the first time during the week that both of us had had the time to sit alone and talk. Our conversation only lasted a short time, since we were both still tired. I started to head back to my room when Leona asked if she could give Dad his morphine instead of me. She said it was something she had to do for her own reasons, and he was due in a few minutes for the next dose. I didn't mind this one time, and said goodnight at four-thirty.

Suddenly, I was awakened by a strong shake on the right arm. It was Leona. "Alberta, wake up. I think Dad just passed away."

I jumped up and ran straight into my parents' bedroom. I glanced first to see where my mother was, discovering her sitting in Dad's rocking chair. She was absolutely still, making no sound at all, staring at him. The low, dim light on the night stand was reflecting a very soft shadow on my father, lying in bed.

I leaned over him and noticed his eyes were open. My heart sank. There was no movement. This was the first time I was in the presence of a person who just passed away. It was terrifying enough, but this was my beloved father. My hands shook as I put them on his chest to feel for any movement. I then placed my hand up to his mouth and nose hoping to feel breath coming from him. There was nothing. I closed his eyes knowing he was gone…Dad was at peace.

Leona explained that after she gave Dad his medicine, she sat in the rocking chair to just share alone time with him in the silence. Moments later, his breathing changed. It wasn't normal. She sensed the worst and walked over to the opposite side of the bed to quietly wake Mom.

As my mother started to sit up, she rubbed both her shoulders. When she did, Dad looked over at her. Leona motioned for Mom to settle down with her in one of the rockers. In case he was dying, Leona wanted no sound around him, so he would go without anyone holding him back. As they sat together, Dad's breathing got worse. He had taken two long, deep breaths then stopped with no further movement.

My insides were trembling as I stood there looking at his body. There was no life in him. He was so still. I started to panic from the reality of it. The control I held for a week was falling apart. Why did he pass away in front of Leona and not me? Why didn't she wake me along with my mother? I selfishly resented not having had this private moment with my father. It was *me* who administered his medicine. This was the one time that I was not by his side. My heart knew deep down, he didn't choose anyone; God just called him. As a daughter, I felt abandoned by him leaving while I slept in the next room.

Leona went to get everyone. They were all sleeping at Joe and Marge's apartment next door. Gradually, all family members came into Dad's bedroom, except Albert. He went straight into the living room. He feared seeing our father. I reminded the family that Dad might still be able to hear us and to tell him we loved him. Leona had a talk with Albert and he eventually approached Dad's bed. We stood around our father, realizing he had left us forever.

Dad passed away on Friday, October 19, 1990 at 5:15 am. Here I was, forty-nine, and I suddenly felt like a child losing all my security. Mom stayed at a distance showing a numb expression on her face. Cathy was called with the news and within minutes she arrived. She called to notify the funeral home. My three brothers had already made the funeral arrangements a few weeks ago so they wouldn't have to be dealt with when the time actually came.

Cathy asked if anyone wanted to help her prepare the body before the funeral home arrived. Light dizziness started to overtake me again. Leona and I wanted our father to keep his dignity while being undressed, so we stepped back. Bill offered and the bedroom door closed.

The funeral director from the Doane, Beal and Ames Funeral Home in North Dennis asked if the family could congregate in another room. He assured us nothing bad would happen, but felt it would be very disturbing if any of us saw the body being removed.

The whole family went up the stairs to the attic on the second floor, except for Bill. He wanted to have some private time alone with Dad. There was nothing for us to sit on, so we just stood standing and waiting. Multiple boxes from the recent move filled the attic. They were scattered, and I wondered if the contents would ever mean anything to Mom again.

We all waited there, feeling odd. The word *body* that was used by the funeral director kept going through my mind. *Removal of the body:* that body was our father! He was somebody. He was ours. He was Brigadier General, Albert L. Gramm, Sr. *Please, don't call him a body.* I wanted to scream, "Refer to him by name!"

I was mad at myself for agreeing to hide upstairs. I had faced everything. Why not this? I felt like my insides were racing. Foolishly, my mind filled with the thought that if I saw him being taken out of the house, it would be easier to face the reality of it. I could hear the director talking at the bottom of the stairs.

For some reason, the attic door unlatched and started to open. It was just enough space for me to catch a glimpse of a shape inside a black zipped-up bag on a gurney. *That was the image the director wanted us to avoid seeing.* I closed my eyes and stepped back. I was warned, and from not listening, I faced a horrible memory. I heard Bill talking to the funeral director and wanted to run down to join him, but my legs were frozen. I could only hear my shallow breathing.

In minutes, the moment for the last farewell was gone. There was enough time to go down the stairs to get a glimpse of the hearse as it pulled out the driveway. In slow motion, it pulled away, leaving me with a separation that was tearing me apart.

Cathy gave her last condolences as we all gathered at the bottom stairway at the front door. It was the same location where Cathy and I had said our first hello. It was only two weeks ago, but it seemed like months. She was about to walk out of our lives and move on to another family needing Hospice services.

Dad had feared dying in a hospital because he considered it a cold place to spend his last days on Earth. I thank God that he got his wish to be at home with all of us. He had the pleasure of seeing our faces every single day at his bedside and to hear our voices and sometimes laughter as we sat with him.

It was so final. The loving care I had given him for the last two weeks of his life had been erased. Dad was no longer in the house and everything was quiet and still in his bedroom. All of us walked around in disbelief not knowing what to say or do. We were so use to being in his bedroom all day. Now, he was gone.

I wanted to console my mother but could feel she was trying to hold herself together. No one was willing to face what had just happened.

I went alone into Dad's bedroom and sat on the edge of the bed where he had lain just an hour ago. The indent from his body was still showing and I rubbed my right hand over the area. His body heat could still be felt under the covers.

He was not going to be there anymore. How was our mother going to stand it? She had been with him for over fifty years. All of us were going to go home and move on the best we could without him. Mom was left with the reality of an absent partner. She had to be in agony.

Leona entered the room and walked over and handed me something. She said, "I think you should have Dad's rosaries along with the prayer book. If you say them every night, in a few weeks you could learn them without reading the book."

His rosaries showed the years of use. There were three cream-colored beads missing from it. I wondered if he rolled them in his fingers during his prayers, and broke them off.

"Since we have been saying the rosaries together," Leona continued, "I want you to know, if they have been under a light for awhile, and you turn the light off, they'll glow in the dark."

No gift could have meant more to me. I thought my presence was going to be a gift to my father, but felt he was leaving me a gift with his death…my faith. It was inside me again and I hungered for it. In my own way, I knew my life was not going to be without God or prayer. I just didn't realize how much of it would be in my daily life.

Leona reached in front of me and took my pillow I had loaned Dad off his bed. She bent down to hand it back to me. "You can have this back now."

That action was the breaking point of my dam. The two weeks of being the strong daughter and sister came to an end. I crunched the pillow into my face, crying with absolutely no control, sobbing and repeatedly saying, "I can still smell him on it! I can still smell him on it!"

The tears just rolled down my checks. Sounds came out of me that I had never known were possible. They were foreign to me. I have cried many times in my life but nothing like this. I felt separated from myself.

No one can understand the pain of losing a beloved parent until you experience it.

My cries were so loud that my mother came rushing down the hallway from the kitchen, still carrying a dish towel over her shoulder. It had been five hours after Dad's death, and she had continued doing the household chores, like nothing had happened.

"Who's crying?" she demanded with an angry face. When she spotted me, she yelled, "Cry your heart out now and *never* cry for your father again! He's at peace." She left the room immediately, so she wouldn't have to console me. If she hadn't left, her strong wall would've collapsed.

She didn't have to explain her request. I knew that it stemmed from her experience with God telling her to let go of Walter. She didn't want my tears to keep our father from going to Jesus.

Now, I knew why my mother had not cried. I finally released my agonizing sorrow from my loss. Time with my father had been good and bad, but I never would've traded any of it. How blessed I was to have spent the last moments of his life with him.

Chapter 21
Facing His Death

My family helped our father move to another world with his life after death. He had become another soul in Purgatory who needed our prayers. This is a place souls go to for purification before they can enter into Heaven. Our Blessed Mother has repeatedly said in her messages to the world, "PRAY, PRAY, PRAY! Souls need our prayers. The deceased can't pray for themselves.

God has a plan for all of us. He gives and He takes. We don't belong to anyone but Him. We are all here for a short time and our lives go by so fast that we don't even see it passing.

At eighty-years old, when Dad was told to get his things in order, he said, "I still have too much left to do." We always think there is time but God calls us with no warning. We have no time to prepare ourselves.

Dad is gone, and I want to become aware of the teachings he was trying to leave for me. I want to follow his belief in compassion, forgiveness, faith; and most of all love. He told me I needed to pay attention to events to be conscious of miracles occurring.

My inner spirituality and faith were reborn after being there for my father's death. It was a lesson for me to realize, we all have to face one last stage of living: dying.

So many times we all turn to God only when we need Him. I realized that material things are not important. The people I love are vital in my life. God keeps trying to tell us, *"Love one another as I have loved you"* *(St. John, 15.12)*. Dad's physical body has left me but his love will live in me through spirit.

Maria returned Friday afternoon, heartbroken that her fear had come true. She missed the last opportunity to be with Dad by a few hours. In reality, all of us said goodbye to him, including her. Once he went into the coma, no one had a chance to say anything to him. If it was left unsaid, it was gone forever.

Cathi Valeriani called the afternoon Dad passed away. She had planned to come and deliver some wonderful news to him. The association was planning a dedication in memory of him. The ceremony was going to be in East Falmouth, right in front of my parents' former home on Fordham Road. They were naming the center island strip the *Al Gramm Park.* Cathi was so heartbroken learning that it was too late to convey this information to him.

The first night without our father fell upon us. The whole family was staying with Mom for the wake and funeral. I had another week before returning to work and could spend the time with her.

I honestly still didn't know how to comfort Mom. My heart kept telling me she didn't want to feel a soft hand on her shoulder or to be embraced. These actions would probably make her fall apart. I was not sure if it was good or bad letting her hold her grief inside for so long.

I entered my bedroom to get undressed and could feel Dad's presence in the next bedroom. It was only this morning I had checked on him in his room. The silence seemed to echo throughout the whole house. No one was in the kitchen talking as we had been for a week.

I felt the loss of Dad and became numb. It was now time to face the reality of his death. *You know it all now, Dad, with the life after! Please God, let him be at peace, forgive him for his sins, and judge him by what was in his heart. He gave so much of himself to all of us. Let him be with Walter.*

I pulled the covers over me, but no position was comfortable. I tossed and turned, only to settle facing the night stand. Dad's rosaries, along with the blue prayer book, were placed on top of it. I took the rosaries in my hands and held them, but my mind couldn't concentrate on praying. My hurt and emptiness were too strong and painful at the moment. As I drifted off to sleep, comfort came from just having them in my possession.

I was abruptly awakened because my body was in the routine of not sleeping very long at a stretch. With all the tension my body was under, I should've passed out until morning. I reached over to switch the light on to see the clock. It showed only a half hour had gone by since I dozed off.

I got out of bed feeling drugged from sleep deprivation. As I crossed the hall to go into the bathroom, I passed by Mom's bedroom. I could hear her tossing and turning, accompanied by soft, deep, moans. I entered her room and did not want to frighten her so I put my hand lightly on her right shoulder.

I bent down and asked her if she was all right. Her back was toward me as she half turned to look up and said, "I don't know what is wrong with me, but I can't sleep!" The tears filled my eyes. *You just lost your husband this morning and you're questioning why you can't sleep?* How alone she must have felt in their bed.

I whispered, "Mom, let me try to help you relax."

I motioned for her to turn over to her side. I reached for the body lotion on her night stand, the same we had used to comfort Dad. I squeezed some out of the tube and proceeded to warm it by rubbing it in my hands before putting it on her back.

As I massaged it into her back muscles, she gave deep sighs. Maybe it was just the motion of being touched and not being alone that brought her comfort. There was no conversation as I continued with slow, firm circular moves spreading the lotion from her neck, shoulders, and down to her lower back and waist. I was glad she was not facing me, because the tears were rolling down my face. I didn't think she had even cried yet. How I ached to hold her and have us cry together.

My mother finally gave a heavy moan and fell asleep. I pulled the warm blankets up to her shoulders and quietly left the room without a word. I returned to my bed, and passed out from complete mental fatigue.

Chapter 22
Planning the Wake

I was awakened Saturday morning with the sun streaming into my room. For a few moments, I lay there and looked out the window, wondering how a day could be so beautiful after such a loss in our lives. I compared it to a hurricane that leaves devastation in its path: once it passes, the bright sunny sky returns, leaving us with only the pieces to pick up.

Everyone assembled into the kitchen to pour their first morning coffee and each was choosing whether to take muffins, donuts or cereal from the counter. We all looked like we were put through a wringer. No one seemed to have the joy or lift to face the day ahead of us. Joe, Albert and Bill had already gone to confirm the final arrangements for the wake and funeral.

Hours later, they returned, with all the preparations completed. Visiting hours would be Sunday from 3:00 pm—5:00 pm and 7:00 pm—9:00 pm at the Doane, Beal and Ames Funeral Home in North Dennis. A funeral Mass would be celebrated at 10:00 am on Monday at Holy Trinity Church in West Harwich. The burial would be at the Massachusetts National Cemetery in Bourne at Otis Air Base.

We all sat down at the kitchen table and four pages were placed on the table that Dad had typed up for us individually before his death. They contained names and phone numbers of who were to be called. He listed family, friends, organizations, associations, including the National Guard service and the Social Security Office. He left Mom information on every single account they had together: credit cards, banks, homeowners and life policies, and in detail the phone numbers to every contact name. All the newspapers were added to the list. Steps on who to see and call after his passing were on the last page. I couldn't believe he did this. We had nothing to look up. He stayed in charge, like the Brigadier General he was, for even his last duties.

Dress clothes for the days ahead were needed. I had not gone home to get any. Al had offered to go to my house and gather up anything that was needed. It seemed like too much hassle to have to explain what to get and from where, so I decided to just go out and buy something. The donations from work would help pay for them.

I went to the plaza a few blocks away from the house and went into the Dress Barn. I chose two white, silky blouses that were really dressy. One was plain and the other had black trim around the collar and sleeves. I ended up with a plain, black, straight polyester skirt.

I walked over to a rack to search for a blazer, in case it got chilly. The weather was still beautiful and it seemed like Indian summer in October. Facing me was a light jacket that had the same shade of black to match everything. I easily found jewelry, so the outfits were completed.

I walked up to the girl at the register with my hands full and placed the items on the counter in front of her. She gave me a warm smile looking through the clothing and replied, "What nice outfits you picked out. Everything is so coordinated. Is it a special occasion?"

I didn't have the heart to embarrass her with the truth of what the occasion was and just answered, "Yes, it is."

A shoe store was next door and a pair of black high heels faced me on the rack. They fit comfortably as I did a trial walk around the store. I grabbed two pair of nylons before cashing out. What a blessing, purchasing everything with no problems. If the items had not fit or matched, I would've broken down on the sidewalk from worrying about completing the last minute details. I grabbed my items and headed back to the house feeling satisfied.

As I entered through the kitchen door, Mom noticed my hands full of bags. "Looks like you got everything you needed," she said with a smile.

She asked to see what was inside the bags, as she tried to take a peek. I gently pulled them away stating it would be a surprise, and placed them in my bedroom.

The newspaper arrived and I sat to look-up the obituaries. Someone else in the family had the responsibility of calling the information in from the list. I couldn't believe the write-up. More shocking, was the fact that Dad wrote it himself. I sat by myself and read the long history about him.

He had joined the 101st Infantry of the Massachusetts National Guard in 1928 and won three National Rifle Association Marksmanship titles during the 1930's. He was inducted into active duty in January of 1941 as a Second Lieutenant. He served in WWII as the commanding officer of the 26th Yankee Division; First Battalion; Company B. For his participation in the Battle of the Bulge, he was decorated with a Bronze Star and was discharged as a Colonel.

After the war, he was involved in the reactivation of the Massachusetts Military Academy. He commanded the Second Battalion of the 104th Infantry Regiment and attained the rank of Brigadier General. He was a graduate and trustee of the Massachusetts Military Academy, graduated from the Army Battalion Commander and Staff Officers School and the Army Command and General Staff College.

It went into memberships to the Lions and Rotary Club, Knights of Columbus, Veterans of Foreign Wars, Retired Officers Association, Secretary to the Ashumet Valley Property Owners, Inc. and church organizations. His civilian positions included being a branch plant manager of Tower Iron Works, assistant to the president of Anderson Aircraft Co., and manager of the Servotronics Division of the Standard-Kollsman Company. He retired as President of Pyrotector, Inc. of Hingham. Through this company he was instrumental in establishing joint ventures and subsidiaries in Germany, Switzerland, England, Australia and Japan.

I took everything in that was written about him. It was the most I knew about my father my whole life. I was learning about him through his obituary. How sad. He had such an interesting and important life and held so many high positions. I felt distressed knowing the multiple questions that I held inside, would never be answered: they went with him.

Chapter 23
The Wake and Funeral

Sunday arrived with the wake facing us. Mom was still holding up. We all gathered at the house waiting for the black, family limos to arrive from the funeral home. Leona's husband, Bob, closed the lumberyard so he could attend. Al was by my side giving me support.

When the two limos arrived, the family filled each car. They backed out of the driveway and my heart started to race. I didn't want to see my father in this state. We drove onto Rte 134 and came upon a traffic light that turned red: it was at the same intersection where I did my shopping the day before.

A car pulled along side of us on our right. I noticed a teenage boy tapping his fingers on the steering wheel to the beat of loud, rap music. The strong vibration could be felt in our limo. He seemed to have no worries in the world. I watched as the other cars rushed in front of us heading down into the plaza. I was amazed. *My father has just died, my world has come apart, and no one notices or cares.*

My life had stopped and I was amazed how the crowds were going about their everyday business with shopping. Nothing disrupted their lives, and they were too busy in their fast-paced world to even look over at us. For a moment, I wished for the impossible; I wanted to bring my father back into my life. It felt like I was never going to be able to laugh and enjoy life again. Was this heavy feeling in my chest ever going to go away? My heart felt as if someone cut it completely out of me.

Within ten minutes, we arrived at the funeral home. Al and I waited for the first car to empty before we entered through the front door. There was this over-powering, fragrance from the mixed flowers. It was one of the realities of being at a funeral home. This time it was not for a friend, it was for my father.

Al and I started to walk toward the casket. I could feel my strength disappearing: my knees felt weak and my body was shaking all over. The closer we got, I started to feel faint. Al took a strong hold of my right arm to support me. An Honor Guard stood tall at the side of the casket with an American flag. We knelt down.

I stared at my father, who looked like a stranger. His features were so dissimilar that I looked around disorientated, thinking we were not in the right room.

"What's wrong?" Al asked.

"I think we have the wrong room. This is not my father."

"It's okay, honey. We are in the right location."

I gazed upon Dad, searching for something familiar. There, on his left shoulder, was an Army rank braided cord insignia, along with his service medals. There was no mistake.

The family blended into a receiving line when people started to arrive. Friends poured past us, not really knowing what to say to comfort us. Instead of our grieving family being consoled, it felt like we were trying to calm the people coming up to us.

I couldn't understand why the tradition stopped for the family members to sit while mourners approached them. It was hard standing a long period of time in such an emotional state. My smile felt pasted on me. My heart was not into greeting anyone. I wanted my heart to heal from this nightmare.

A stranger in the line was now facing me. The gentleman looked to be in his late seventies and held himself proudly. He gently took my hand and introduced himself as John Hamilton. He was from Iowa and had served under my father during WWII. His eyes filled when he mentioned the events they shared together and stated he never forgot him. With sadness, he described how bad the cold, freezing winters were fighting during WWII.

"The military had problems keeping up with food rations for the regiments. Your father saw to it; no matter what was happening during the battles or where we were, he had a meal delivered to us every single day, even if it was a small portion. He was a great and wonderful man. I'm proud to have served under him."

I held his hand and thanked him for taking such a long trip to say goodbye to Dad. The story was short because others behind him waited to pass to the next family member. I watched as he sat in the front row, facing my father. His eyes never left him even with all the turmoil going on. Nothing broke his concentration. John had gone up to the casket and touched the insignia on my father's shoulder.

I had tried to stay polite as friends were coming up to me showing their sympathy, but my eyes searched in between the line to watch for John. The physical openness from his grief only added to my own sorrow. He had sat back down in the same chair, facing Dad. I couldn't concentrate on anyone talking to me.

John had positioned his elbows on his knees, and placed his head into his hands. I watched as his broad shoulders shook. I had not missed seeing the devotion, respect and love from his gaze at my father. He straightened up, and ran his fingers through his gray hair. I saw him wipe his eyes with his handkerchief, as he leaned back into the chair.

I told myself that when the lines thinned out, I'd go over and talk to him to learn more about my dad's life. I wanted to get his phone number so we could finish our conversation. He sat there entranced, as though reliving the memories and experiences.

The mourners came in large groups and completely blocked my view of the man. When the lines slowed down, I looked for the ex-soldier. He was gone without me having had a chance to join him. The chance to know all those stories went with the stranger. He could have been one of the closest men to Dad during the war. Even to this day, I long to revive that moment with him.

I have learned that time waits for no one. The important things have to come first, because if you hesitate, they disappear. A group from the

Knights of Columbus arrived and lined-up in front of the casket to say prayers. Seeing them in their uniforms and standing so proud was touching. The respect for my father from everyone there made me very proud of him.

I glanced in a corner only to notice Joe St. Onge standing away from the crowd all alone in the shadows. I walked up and hugged him. His body was trembling. I asked him if he had been up to see my father yet. He'd not been able to do it.

"Joe, would you like me to go up with you?"

He looked relieved. "I'd appreciate that. I can't go alone."

I wrapped my arm through his and we both walked toward Dad. We knelt in prayer as Joe wept. How glad I was to have seen him before he walked out without saying his final farewell.

After the wake, friends and family came to the house. I watched Mom as she sat far in a corner by herself. People were talking and laughing, without any of them taking the time to acknowledge her personally. Funny how people outside the family, seemed to act like nothing had really happened. I know life will go on for everyone but it had stopped for Mom.

The funeral was upon us Monday morning…the final day. This would be our last chance to physically see our father. I entered the funeral home and sat in front to absorb every feature of Dad for a lifetime. It seemed so unreal. After prayers were said by the priest, people were called to line-up in their cars for Mass. I walked up to Dad and placed my hand on his. I couldn't bring my tears to the surface. I still felt like I was in shock.

When we arrived at church, the Honor Guard was already standing outside along with the Knights of Columbus members. The Gulf War was going on and we were lucky to get an Honor Guard for the wake and funeral. They lent an impressive military atmosphere and it was heartwarming to see Dad's military status being recognized.

Seeing the men in their uniforms made me feel the absence of Dad even more. I pictured my father alone side of them. So many years, he had attended the National Guard meetings in uniform.

The sight of them lined up so proudly, brought me back to the day when Dad had taken me to a Memorial Day parade in Rhode Island. I was around twelve years old at the time.

We had arrived early to reserve a spot on the street so no one would block our view of the parade. As the different organizations, floats, and school bands passed by us, an Army unit could be seen approaching. I didn't know at the time that it was the 101st Infantry of the 26th Yankee Infantry Division or that Dad had been their commanding officer during WWII. They marched directly in front of us.

The Army's military band followed right behind them. The marching soldiers were ahead of the band, just far enough so the instrumental sounds were at a distance. The rhythm of the shuffling feet of the soldiers could be heard when their boots hit the pavement. They marched in perfect unison and every step was in sequence with the each other's. They stood proud and tall with their eyes straight ahead. The soldiers' demeanors exemplified their pride in wearing the uniforms with honor.

As the Army band came closer, the overriding sounds started to descend upon us. The drums and horns vibrated deep in my chest and ears as well as under my feet as I stood on the sidewalk.

The whole atmosphere gave me a sense of distinguished military men. It was a wonderful experience as I witnessed a branch of the military trying to show civilians how proud they are to protect this country. Even at a young age, I understood this.

I looked up at Dad to say something to him, while the group was still proceeding by us. I saw something I'd never forget. There was my father, in his plain, weekend clothes, standing tall saluting the unit going by while tears rolled down his checks. He stood just as proud as each officer who marched by.

Back then, being young, I thought Dad was being sentimental thinking about the memories when he was in the service. Now, as an adult, I understand more clearly the pain my father probably felt with the recollections of his fallen comrades. It must've been heartbreaking for him to remember the soldiers who didn't come home. He had been in charge of making serious decisions for the servicemen in his unit.

It had been the first time, as a child, that I saw my father cry. Seeing him in such an uncontrollable state scared me. I'd grown up feeling security because he had been so strong with his emotions. He never showed any weakness. I had seen a different side of him. To this day, when I hear a military band, it chokes me up. I go back, to that moment in time, with Dad saluting.

The family started to assemble and go down the church aisle. My eye caught Trisha, my manager from work, and Roberta sitting on the right side. It warmed my heart knowing they drove an hour and a half to be there.

We were ushered to the front pew as the Knights of Columbus members wheeled the casket up front with the American Flag draped over it. As Mass was being said, my mind absorbed nothing. Deep in my heart, I knew God was giving all of us tremendous strength. Every one of us had been in complete control without any expression of grief. When Mass ended, I walked outside to thank Trisha for coming. She gave me her condolences and explained she had to return back to the office. Roberta planned to come to the cemetery and brunch so she joined in the car procession.

One by one, people entered their cars to go to Otis Air Base. The Massachusetts National Cemetery is located in Barnstable County on Cape Cod, approximately 65 miles southeast of Boston and adjacent to the Otis Air Force Base.

As we ascended a hill on Route 6, I looked back through the rear window of the funeral limo. It was shocking to see the number of cars with their headlights on that followed the motorcade. The family had been blessed with so many friends coming to bid farewell to Dad.

The cars entered at a crawl through the entrance of the black, heavy iron gates of the cemetery. *Oh Lord, I don't want to be here.* The limo parked near an open section with chairs lined up under a canopy on the lawn. It was completely apart from the grave site. Seven servicemen with rifles along with two Honor Guards got out of an Army van to stand at parade rest.

The casket was placed on top of a high stand in front of the family and draped again with the American flag. I looked over to my right at my mother. She looked pale. *How was she holding herself together— how were all of us?* I hadn't witnessed one person break down since Dad had passed away.

After the priest gave the blessings, he walked over to my mother. He bent down and whispered something to consol her. Without any warning, the seven servicemen had started a rifle squad salute by firing three rounds. It's a military honor for a veteran. My whole body jumped from the over-powering, loud explosions from the rifles. *Oh God! My insides are coming apart. I'm not going to make it.* As each shot rumbled through the hillside, it echoed deep within my chest. I could feel the emotions buried inside me trying to escape. I bit my lip as the moisture in my eyes blurred my vision. Two Honor Guards took the flag off the casket and started to fold it in the proper military manner.

When they concluded, one of the soldiers started toward my mother and gently placed the flag into her hands. I looked at her and saw a defeated women acting with pride. My heart ached for her. I knew she was not really this strong. My love for her was even stronger knowing the battle she was fighting with emotions.

At this point, I expected my mother to totally break down. Instead, she sat up straight, the proud wife of a Brigadier General. The pain in my throat was choking me. *Please, God, hold me together a little longer.* All of us could not comfort one another because each person would have collapsed. We were determined not to shed a tear publicly. We were military children and wanted to honor our father.

The service ended quickly and everyone started to walk away to their cars to attend the brunch on the Army base. Al sensed I needed this time to say goodbye to Dad, so he mixed into the crowd leaving.

I was the only one left sitting in my chair. I walked over to the casket and put my head down on it and cried.

"Oh, Dad, I'm so sorry. If only I had taken the time to know you completely. Please forgive me. I had so much to tell you. I love you, I love you."

This was the last private moment with my father.

I don't remember the buffet, or if I even ate anything. I just remember looking at the tables filling so fast and asking Leona where Dad was going to sit. We looked at each other with disbelief of my mind lapse. I couldn't fathom something like that coming out of my mouth. It had been a miracle that we both held up.

The brunch lasted about an hour, and people started to thin out saying their goodbyes. The family members made their way to the limos and were dropped off at the house. This was my last connection to my father. We were left with our memories.

Again, we became hosts for our very close friends and family as they entered the kitchen where sandwiches, desserts and coffee were waiting. I sat there silently, as I watched everyone laughing and having loud conversations. When the last person left, we were wiped out, and avoided speaking about the tragedy.

I had another week to spend with Mom and the events during this time are totally blank in my memory. For some reason, the weeks of Dad's illness and death were clear, but not the week afterward.

I do remember spending days in Mom's bedroom wanting to be alone. There I would sit and rock in the over-sized rocker facing Dad's bed. My imagination drifted back until I could picture him lying there. The bad moments were good: at least then, he had still been in my life.

Chapter 24
Getting on with Life

The time arrived for me to go home and take on the everyday responsibilities of home life and working. Mom was left in the hands of Joe and Marge. Dad died knowing she would always be loved and be well taken care of by the two of them. I would no longer be making phone calls nor having visits watching him run around the house fixing things. There would be no more pulling out of the driveway, looking back, and seeing my father waving goodbye to me. Now life without him would be only memories.

Dad told me numerous times family was the most important thing in life. I remember his saying that a home is where you make it and not to fear the change of a new move. He advised me never to be scared to take a chance, because with change, you grow. If you fail at something, just get up and start over again. He explained with each time he moved the change was always for bigger and better positions. If he hadn't made the changes, the family would not have had the things he gave us.

I went back to work, knowing my heart was not ready to deal with the everyday problems of customers complaining on the phone. The pain of losing my father was still fresh in my soul. I tried to work while fighting the depression. I just wanted to be by myself outside of work. It is not often that bosses sit and wait for their employers to pull themselves together. They have a business to run and money to make.

I sat at my desk doing my job day after day with an empty feeling inside of me. It was as if time had stopped.

On November 29, 1990, Bill and Sharon had a baby girl they named Olivia. Her birth occurred five weeks after Dad's passing. It was so close, and yet so far. It was not the boy our father thought would arrive, but two years later on April 13, 1992, they would have a son, Brandon—another grandson to carry on the Gramm name.

Dad was thrilled Bill and Sharon were having a baby because they didn't want a family in the beginning. Bill was in his forties and surprised my father with the news. Before Dad died, he was blessed with knowing they would have a child. He would've been so proud and happy to have little feet running around the house again. He had wished for more grandchildren to be added to the family.

A few weeks before Christmas, Joe and Marge had informed the family that Mom was bedridden with bronchitis. After work, I had made the trip to South Dennis to see her.

Being wintertime, it was already dark out when I arrived. Unlike the other houses in the neighborhood, the outside of my parents' house had no Christmas lights to brighten up the yard. It seemed so eerie. Christmastime had always been a big holiday in our family, even as grown-ups. We had always laughed with embarrassment about how many presents were always under the tree: here we were adults, and we had more presents than most children.

It was not that way this time. When I had entered through the kitchen door, Joe greeted me and said Mom had been on medication but didn't look good. As I started down the hall to her bedroom, I glanced towards the living room. What an empty sight. There stood their Christmas tree: bare, with no lights or decorations. There was not a single gift under the tree. I walked into the room and stood staring at the misplaced tree. It was worse to see it there than to not have one at all. Dad's death filled the house. Everything had stopped: not only our lives, but our spirit.

I continued my journey down the hall to see Mom. She was lying in bed, the same one she had shared with Dad. It was not that long ago that I came to see him. I bent down to kiss her and sat on the edge of the bed.

She was surprised to see me on a weeknight. "What are you doing here?"

"I missed you and thought I'd take a ride to see how you're doing. Joe said you were not feeling well," I said.

"No, I'm not," she replied.

Mom looked gray. I feared she was dying and was going to leave us two months after my father. I placed my hand on her forehead to see if she felt hot. She did not seem to have a fever.

I watched her closely as she talked and moved in bed. Mom did not look like she had a serious condition.

"How are you really doing, Mom?"

Tears started to fill her eyes. "If only I could make a year, I'd be alright." A year was so far off.

I held her hand. She was physically sick from the loss of her husband. Mom's expression showed she could care less about what happened to her. Nothing gave her excitement, happiness, or even the will to go on. My heart ached for her. I let her cry and talk about Dad to clear the pain out of her empty heart.

At least my visit had given her some comfort. She had the opportunity to express her grief and loneliness with someone to listen.

Chapter 25
Spiritual Signs

I was about to discover the many spiritual gifts left to me, even the ones before Dad's death. The power of the Holy Spirit was stronger than I could ever have imagined. It just took my father's passing to make me aware of them. Now, everything was starting to fall into place.

So many mystical events had and were about to enter my life. I thought about when Albert had introduced the Medjugorje tapes to the family. He said there was a newspaper, published by a Wayne Weible, who wrote about these events and that one could obtain a monthly subscription. Leona and I had taken the address, intending to subscribe. I remembered that when Dad was sick, he wanted to go to Medjugorje, but the cancer had made him too weak to do any traveling. I was still not practicing my faith, but strongly believed in God and these apparitions. As usual, I became too busy and forgot all about the paper or events for years.

On June 2, 1991, seven months after my father's death, the Ashumet Valley Property Owners, Incorporated, in conjunction with the Town of Falmouth, had the dedication for Dad. The main entrance parcel of the Ashumet Valley was named the *Al Gramm Park*. It was in Dad's memory for his many years being their Secretary with invaluable service to the association. Cathi Valeriani, Vice President, came to present Mom with a plaque.

Our whole family, including the grandkids and our grandmother, shared in the day's event. Mom's mother was ninety-five years old and we were fortunate that she had the health to join us. Chairs were placed on the center island directly in front of their former home on the corner of Fordham Road and Route 151 in East Falmouth. It was a very emotional and proud time for all of us.

After the ceremony, we had a family cookout across the street, in the backyard of my parents' former home. It was almost a year since the move to South Dennis and the house was still not sold. It felt so strange to walk through the vacant house and reminisce about all the memories. When a loved one is missing, a place can be so meaningless. The emptiness resonated in the deepest part of me. It was more painful returning than staying away.

In May of 1993, I was finally scheduled to have a hysterectomy to remove my fibroid tumors. It was held off for seven years and I could not wait any longer. I was having my surgery at the Brigham and Women's Hospital in Boston. The night before, Al was in my living room in Dighton watching television, while I was in my bedroom, packing my clothes neatly into the suitcase.

At the time, I had no particular thoughts going through my mind except trying to remember everything that would be needed for the five-day stay. Silly as it may sound, I was actually looking forward to being spoiled: getting three meals a day placed in front of me and having time to read a book or to say my rosary, privately, everyday. Those crazy wishes showed me how seldom I took time for myself.

I was trying not to think about the actual surgery because the fear of it would put me in a complete panic. I wanted so much to be brave in front of Al. At the age of fifty-two, I didn't want to act like a child.

From out of nowhere, I heard this voice say, "Do not be afraid. I'll be with you." This voice did not come from someone near me but I heard it *inside* my head. At that very second, a current—an indescribably strong feeling—entered directly through the outside of my head and went through my whole body. I felt it enter through my skull and it caused no pain. It traveled with a speed I never knew could exist. It took only one to two seconds for it to happen.

This feeling rushed instantly from my head to every part of my inner body and touched every nerve-ending, even to the end of my fingers and toes. It spread in one fast sweep until it hit every limb, adding an immediate calmness and peace over me.

I stood there, in complete wonder and shock. *What just happened to me? What did I experience?* This voice hit the deepest part of my brain. I knew in my heart that this was a spiritual experience. I stood there motionless; remembering only a peaceful, soft, male voice. I thought back to when my mother heard God and knew it was now my experience.

I don't know why I didn't tell Al what happened to me immediately after the event. *How could I explain it?* I was afraid he would think I was under a lot of stress before my operation.

I went to bed that night without taking a tranquilizer. When I had other surgeries, my heart would pound with fright so bad that I would be up all night. All negative thoughts would run through my mind on what *could* go wrong. This time, sleep came to me with ease and not once did I wake up.

Morning came and we were on the road at four in the morning traveling to the hospital. We had to arrive by six. Al and I talked and laughed the whole hour, without me even thinking about the surgery. When we arrived at the hospital, I joked with the nurses and the anesthesiologist while I was waiting to be wheeled into the operating room. There was nothing but absolute calmness in me and it had to be the most peace I have ever been conscious of.

I somehow pushed the experience to the back of my mind and didn't talk about it to anyone. I simply acknowledged it and didn't try to analyze it. I would think about it from time to time, but it seemed like an event that should be kept to myself.

It was not until months later, when Al and I were watching a special program on television, that I vocalized the event. People who had had spiritual experiences were being interviewed. A soldier told a story of his being inside an Army tank during the Korean War. He had been frightened for his life when he heard a voice tell him, "Do not be afraid. You will not die!" Then he described the same wave I had experienced, going through his body and giving him the same peace. It was then that I told Al my story of what happened to me before my surgery.

On September 23, 1993, Al and I were married to add to our spiritual blessings. After ten years being together, we said our vows in St. Rose of Lima Church in Rochester. It was a simple and private candlelight wedding during a week night. Al didn't want anyone to know about it, including our children. He didn't want to make a big event out of it since we were together for so long.

I was uncomfortable omitting our six kids. We were extremely fortunate that they all loved each other and both Al and I. I agreed as long as we were married in the church.

There were shocked reactions and disappointments from the family. It didn't take long for the excitement to spread and all was forgiven. Everyone respected our decision and held no bad feelings against us. Both families had been happy that we all had become one big family.

My home in Dighton was sold and I moved to Rochester. It was a small country town with beautiful fields and farm land. I loved it from the first time I traveled through it.

Al's oldest son, Alan, was single, and in his early forties. Lynne was in her late thirties, married, and had a son. Carol and John were still single, in their early twenties, and still living at home. My daughters, Debbie and Lori were both married, in their twenties, and had two children each. We were fortunate that all six got along very well and they all loved each other.

Columbus Day was arriving and my girlfriend, Rita Vasconcellous, from Westport, had invited me to go to her cousin's home in Lake George, NY, for the long weekend, with five other friends. My girlfriend, Roberta, from work was tagging along with the group. Al's son, Alan, had tickets to see the Boston College football team play in Michigan and had invited Al to go with him. It was perfect timing to fill my weekend without him.

The trip was worth taking just for the scenery alone. It was beautiful. On our way, we stopped at a rest area surrounded by mountains. The girls brought a "roadside" gourmet picnic of wine and shrimp. We placed a plastic table cover on a picnic table and with a few laughs, good food and an hour's relaxation, we were ready for the balance of the traveling time.

Rita's cousins' home had four bedrooms upstairs and additional sleeping quarters downstairs. We spent our nights, playing cards to the wee/early hours of the morning. One afternoon we went to small country town for a day of just shopping and browsing; a very favorite activity of most women.

Doris, a girl from our group, and I entered an antique shop while the others continued on into different stores on the street. I noticed a huge, old beer barrel that was filled to the top with holy medals. There were hundreds of medals to choose from in every size, shape, and color. I had been searching for years to find a special one of the Blessed Mother.

There it was…so different. The medal was oval and gold plated with the outside scalloped with a silver trim. In the center, it had the figure of Our Lady in silver. No necklace…just the pendant. The sign above the barrel said, "A dollar."

A dollar! It must be junk. I turned it over, only to see the name *Jerusalem* inscribed in the center of it. *Jerusalem…a medal made in Jerusalem.* I felt closer to Our Lady knowing it came from there.

How can I go wrong for a dollar? The worst that can happen is it turns black and I'll have to get rid of it. Another woman was watching me like a hawk patiently waiting and hoping for me to put it down. Her continuous stare at the medal I was holding, was what got me moving to the cash register really fast. I held onto the medal like it was a piece of jewelry bought at Tiffany's until it was paid for at the counter. The pendant is still with me all these years, and it has never tarnished, even though I wear it in the shower.

My mother gave me my father's gold necklace he wore everyday. Connected to it was a tiny, blue medal of the Blessed Mother that Dad cherished. I added my medal to his necklace. It gave me a great sense of closeness to my father. It is very rare that it comes off me.

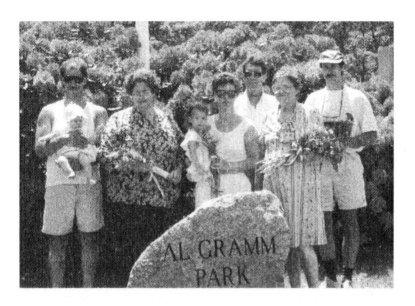

Left: Bill, Leona, Alberta, Mom/Back left: Albert & Joe

Chapter 26
An Apparition

Not long after my trip to New York, Joe called me to say Mom fell in the shower and was being rushed to the Cape Cod Hospital in Hyannis. He was sure she'd had a stroke because there was no movement on one side of her face and she was having trouble talking.

After her examination, the doctors confirmed a stroke and decided to have her transferred to the Joslin Clinic in Boston. I traveled an hour after work three times a week to see her. Roberta accompanied me on my first visit, knowing I was upset with the news.

Upon entering the hospital room, I expected to see Mom with serious physically changes from the stroke. She had no problem speaking and I was thankful there was only a slight paralysis on the right side of her face.

In addition to Mom being diabetic for years, the stroke had weakened her vision. She was now seeing double with the right eye and her right hand was shaking constantly. My mother was facing months of rehabilitation. She remained in the hospital for three weeks and because her legs were now unsteady, she had to use a walker to get around.

It was not long after that, she had cataract surgery in both eyes, leaving her disappointed and frustrated because there was no difference in her sight. Being seventy-nine years old, diabetic, and having had a stroke, didn't help her eyesight. She wore a patch over her weak eye to keep from seeing double.

In 1996, I heard about a nun claiming to have seen the Blessed Mother in Medway, Massachusetts. Leona and I decided to take our mother to pray over her. We had hoped a blessing would happen and she would regain some of her sight or hearing. This holy place was not yet acknowledged by the Catholic Church, even after miracles were received by pilgrims who had made trips there. A person could easily ride right by the location because there were no large signs indicating what was in this area. It was just an open field with a path going into the woods.

Friends had informed us that the site was on Rte 126 in Medway. We were told to ride very slowly and watch for an old, broken down, wooden fence on our right with a gate askew and leaning on the ground. Next to it was a small scratched white sign that said *Betania.* We finally found it and Leona parked the car on the side of the road at the entrance gate on the main highway.

It was in the middle of October with an unusually cold rawness in the air, causing us to wear our heavy winter coats that day. We placed Mom in her wheelchair and wrapped a warm wool blanket across her lap and legs. Leona and I buttoned our coats close to our necks.

We crossed the open field until we came to a dirt path that led through a group of trees in the woods. It was not long before we came upon a tiny wooden bridge. The stream running under it was very shallow, almost dried up. The sight of the water only made the air seem colder, and a chill went right through me.

It was so peaceful; the only sound came from the wind going through the trees. Blue crosses were placed in locations where people claimed to have seen Our Lady. The path suddenly branched out in different directions, confusing us as to which way to go. At the intersection, a huge boulder had holy statues placed on top of it. Pilgrims who had been there had left letters, family portraits, rosaries, and holy articles all over the massive rock and on the surrounding tree branches around it.

There were only a few leaves exposed on the trees because of the fall foliage and high wind storms. The loss of leaves left the area open, displaying the multiple paths we could choose to follow. We started to understand why no one else was there that day, since there was no protection from the cold.

The three of us decided to travel up the path on our left. We could see a picnic table with two large statues of St. Joseph and The Blessed Mother behind it. This was the only section that appeared to have a place for Mom to sit and be comfortable while we prayed.

As we started toward the area, we noticed the ground was wet and muddy from the last storm. The wheelchair had to be abandoned three quarters of the way up the path because it was sinking into the soft ground. Leona and I couldn't budge it. We both supported my mother under her arms and helped her walk to the table.

After settling Mom, we noticed another deeper stream nearby. I had heard stories about people taking water from it and being healed from their illnesses. We had brought plastic gallon milk jugs and started filling them with what we believed to be holy water.

We went back to join Mom at the table and noticed she already had her rosary beads out. We were only there a few minutes when she needed to use a restroom. Directly across from us on the other side of the path, maybe fifteen to twenty feet, was a small shed, which I hoped had a restroom in it.

I supported her by the hand as we walked across to the shed. The windows had wood across them so I couldn't see what was inside the building. I completed a full walk around it, hoping to see a door so we could enter. The building was locked up completely and I was now faced with what to do for her. It would take too much time and distance if we headed back to the car and drove her somewhere. The next step was to find out if the three of us were alone in the area. People were always arriving to pray. I didn't want to be surprised by anyone coming upon us unexpectedly and embarrassing my mother. So far, we were the only ones in the area.

With the section being entirely wide open, I could see all the way down the path we had just come up. There was no one in sight. The entrance was also visible, and if someone was coming, we would have plenty of time to spot them. Three sides of the shed were surrounded by marshland, so no one could come through it. We were totally alone in this area. There was only one way in and one way out.

Leona was across the path sitting at the picnic table, and watched in case she spotted a new arrival. My sister yelled back to me that no one was anywhere in sight. It took only twenty seconds for Mom to complete her task. Out of the blue, a woman *stepped* from around the corner of the tiny shed only a few feet from us. You have to understand…I had just walked around the shed and no one had been there! There was only one path that she could have taken to get to our location. And, Leona would've seen her.

When the three of us traveled up the path, leaves, branches and twigs were all over the ground and our boots made a crunching sound when we had walked over the debris. Our movement had echoed through the woods so no one could have possibly walked through it without making any noise. Not one sound was heard from her approaching, and she was not there when I looked earlier.

The woman walked right by me and headed straight toward my mother. It was like I was utterly invisible. Not once did she look embarrassed or shocked, knowing why we were at the shed. As the stranger reached out to balance my mother by the elbow, she asked, "Can I help you?" The woman, without waiting for a reply from my mother, proceeded to lead her back to the picnic table toward Leona with me following behind. *How did she even know my mother was handicapped and needed help?*

Mom's mouth dropped open, wondering who this woman was and where she had come from. A person does not ordinarily come up to a stranger and throw herself on them. Leona had the same shocked expression as we approached. The woman helped Mom sit down at the table, while I questioned Leona as to what direction this woman had come from when we both had confirmed no one was in the area.

My sister answered, "This woman *didn't* come up that path. I was watching the whole time. She didn't come from anywhere…*she just appeared.*"

The woman placed herself at our table without an invitation and said, "My name is Miriam and I come here to help people pray." She looked to be in her early forties and was soft spoken. There was a very peaceful way about her. She was dressed no differently than anyone coming into the woods and was wearing a pair of slacks and a warm coat.

Leona sat across from Mom. Miriam was directly opposite of me. She asked if we wanted to say the rosary with her.

My mother, who is always outspoken, answered, "We can say our own." She was upset that this woman forced herself on us and was not leaving.

I was starting to feel differently because it seemed something was going on, but I didn't understand what it was at the time. There was no conversation from Miriam like strangers normally have when you first meet. She didn't care to know anything about us…nothing. It honestly felt like she had been expecting us and was waiting.

Miriam reached over the picnic table and took my hands, asking me to join her in prayer. She never took her eyes off me as she talked, or even acknowledge Mom or Leona.

Her stare went directly into my heart making me feel so much peace and love that I can't begin to describe it. Mom and Leona finally joined hands with us. The two large statues of Mary and St. Joseph were directly behind us.

Miriam started saying the *Our Father* and *Hail Mary* and we proceeded to follow along with her. I closed my eyes to concentrate hard for Jesus to hear my request for my mother. Then a strong feeling came over me to pray; not just by saying words, but to feel it from the heart.

While my eyes were still shut, I automatically took over and repeated one prayer right after another without stopping. I was so filled with emotion that it actually caused me to cry and tears started flowing down my face.

I was so immersed in the feeling of love, and so deep in prayer, that I lost the feeling of being on Earth. When my eyes opened, I had to remind myself where I was. My body felt like it had been floating and there was no connection to anyone at the table.

I looked up at the trees and the leaves were all in a very vibrant gold. I gazed upon the two statues and their faces where encircled with haloes of golden glow. I cried out to everyone, "Look. Everything's gold!"

They turned to study the space. Neither of them could see what I saw. Leona said she saw some gold on Mom's right hand which had been damaged by the stroke.

Miriam never once took her eyes off me or turned around to see what I was talking about; which would have been the normal thing to do.

I looked across to see Miriam's reaction, only to find she was staring directly at me with a smile of satisfaction. She was not the least bit shocked or interested in what I was witnessing. All this time, she continued to look only at me. From her continuous stare, I had no doubt she already knew this was going to happen. I found it odd, she didn't want to mentioned the event or talk about it.

Her smile went right through me and I sensed a great love from her. The connection was so strong, I would have spent a long time praying with her had I been alone. There was a mystery all around her. She hadn't been surprised that I saw gold in the trees.

Miriam didn't say the rosary. That was supposed to be the reason for her being there. Once I witnessed the gold, she got up and said she had to leave. She went over to my mother and gave her a hug before leaving. Her presence only lasted about ten or fifteen minutes.

The three of us sat in silence as we watched Miriam start her walk down the path we had come up. She stopped at Mom's wheelchair, looked up at the sky, and then lifted her arms up high like she was praying to God. We watched her in complete wonder, trying to understand what she was doing.

At this *exact* moment, Leona's rosaries fell off the picnic table. When she bent down to pick them up from the ground, our attention went away from Miriam.

We watched Leona pick up the rosaries, and in *seconds,* looked back again to see what Miriam was doing. *She was gone!* There was no possible way she could have gone down the path that fast. The trail was too long. Miriam disappeared as suddenly as she had arrived.

Mom looked at the two of us and asked, "What just happened? What did we just witness?" The three of us knew what had just happened was an act from Heaven.

Leona then said to me, "Do you know who Miriam is?"

I replied, "No, who?"

She choked up and said, "Miriam is the name of Our Blessed Mother Mary in Hebrew!"

"Leona, are you saying you believe that was our Blessed Mother?"

"Alberta, what just happened to us was not normal."

"I won't even argue that point. Something spiritual happened. This woman wasn't from Earth. The visionaries had always claimed Our Lady appeared to them as she really is so I truly believe we had had an encounter with an angel," I remarked.

That would explain the feelings I was having during the prayers. One hears about these appearances, but we don't ever expect to experience them. We were specially blessed. Dad told me to open my eyes to things happening around me and this was one of those days. It was a miracle never to be explained, but only witnessed as a gift from above.

Our strange phenomena had been one of many apparitions at Medway. Other pilgrims, who had visited the shrine, had claimed the sun would spin and turn colors or had witnessed the same gold throughout the wooded area. A blue cross is placed wherever someone had witnessed an apparition with Our Lady.

In September of 1998, another blessed event happened at the same location. Maria Esperanza, who had been considered to be one of the greatest mystics of our time, went to the same shrine in Medway to pray with her husband, George, and other members of the Bianchini family. She believed in the existence of realities beyond human comprehension through apparitions with God.

Maria lived in Venezuela and often had stigmata; which is bleeding of the hands. Stigmata are wounds or marks on a person resembling the five wounds (two hands, the feet, and in his side) received by Jesus at the crucifixion. Maria told the staff of the Marian Messengers in

Medway that when she arrived in front of the Statue of Our Lady, something beautiful happen to her.

While she was praying, Jesus appeared to her and said, "Tell members of the Marian Community that they need to build some kind of protection for the Image of My Mother on the land at Medway. Her image needs to be protected from the elements. When this is done, My Mother will open her arms wide and embrace those who come to pray and give them new hope."

Sister Margaret from the Marian Community contacted Mr. James Merloni, the coordinator for the Labormen's Working Camp in Hopkinton to inquire about building a grotto on the land. In less than three weeks, the grotto was completed thanks to Mr. and Mrs. James Merloni, their son, James and Mr. Ray Conti, the stone mason who came out of retirement to build "Our Lady's Protection."

On October 20, 1998, Fr. Tom DilLorenzo, blessed the grotto in Medway. Ivan, one of the six visionaries from Medjugorje, in Bosnia had attended the blessing and had his daily apparition at the grotto site with Our Lady. Ivan married a girl from Boston and lives six months out of the year here in the United States to be close to his wife's family.

It goes to prove there is something very mystical with this location. That may have been the reason the three of us were completely alone in shrine area.

Chapter 27
Searching for Material on Medjugorje

After having had this experience in Medway, and nine years after Albert introduced me to Medjugorje, I began to long for any book about this little village. I felt a power beyond my control was calling me to do this. Too many things were happening in my life that couldn't be explained. I wanted to learn as much as possible about the apparitions of Our Lady seen by the six children.

The desire to have God in my life was stronger than ever. I started to become conscious of the fact that He waits patiently and lovingly for souls to turn to Him. When I opened myself up completely to God during Dad's illness, I was coming into my own spirituality. I *wanted* God in my life, and begin to realize, He *was* my life.

I was slowly renewing my religious beliefs. Our parents brought all of us up as Catholics and encouraged us to practice it. Once we married and moved out on our own, many of us stopped practicing our faith. They worried because their children turned away from church. Not living at home any longer, we had found excuses on why we couldn't give an hour to God. Maybe their prayers were being answered. Leona and I were the only ones returning to our church. My brothers, for some reason, never had the slightest desire or felt the need.

Now my mother, Leona and I have picked up where Dad left off praying for the rest of the family to convert by turning back to Mass and confession. How lucky I am to have time left in my life to make the changes to turn my life around. I wanted to learn as much as possible what Our Lady was asking of us.

For close to a year after Dad's death, Leona went to church every single morning before work to pray for his soul. She knew our father feared suffering in Purgatory after fighting in WWII. While attending one Mass, total peace came over her. She knew at that very moment he was okay. She felt it was God's way of saying, "He is with Me now," so she let go. She put her trust in God that Dad was in Heaven.

One Sunday, Leona and I decided to go to the LaSalette Shrine in Attleboro for confession and to just meditate. We were always close and shared our faith; we could talk about our religion for hours. I wanted Al to join us, but he had no interest in going to shrines or Mass.

He said, "Alberta, go and pray. It's not my thing."

When I started going back to church myself, I prayed constantly for him to convert. He believed in his faith but did not want to put the effort out to practice it. All the time we dated, the both of us never went to church. We had lost our way. When I attended Mass at St. Rose of Lima in Rochester, I would see couples together, and ached for Al to be with me. I came home from Mass one time and told him someone was asking for him.

Being surprised, he said, "Really, who?"

I replied with a smile, "God!"

The guilt strategy and humor did not work. He told me continuously he believed and didn't need to go to church. Al felt confession was between him and God and there was no need to go to a priest for forgiveness.

My sister and I made our trip to LaSalette Shrine together. She closed her lumberyard in Buzzard Bay for the day. Her husband, Bob, was now running their furniture business in Punxsutawney, PA. That's where their original home was located.

After we went to confession, lit candles, and prayed, we headed straight to the gift store. We went our separate ways in the book section, searching out what interested each of us.

I was amazed how much was written on Medjugorje. It made me

feel like I'd had my head buried in sand for years about this event. I didn't know which book to pick up first. Then in front of me, was *Medjugorje the Message,* by Wayne Weible. I picked it up and read through some of the pages. The pictures inside were the selling point for me. I wanted to see what the little town looked like, along with the visionaries. I went up to the counter with other religious articles along with my book. We spent the rest of the day walking the grounds.

I came home with the excitement of wanting to jump right into reading my book. I waited until after supper and got comfortable in the corner of the couch with my pillow and picked up my book. Just looking at the cover with the name *"Medjugorje"* made my heart leap. The anticipation of turning the first page was worth waiting for. I knew in my heart this book was not only going to be special but important.

Page after page had me so mesmerized that I couldn't put it down. I grabbed onto every word, pictured every event and location, and studied each visionary's life. I just felt like I belonged there.

It would be eleven in the evening before I realized it was time for bed. I knew when the alarm went off in the morning I would be tired for work. After shutting the light off and pulling the covers over me, I went into a deep sleep, dreaming of this little village on the other side of the world.

I spent every single evening reading my book on the couch. I tried imagining making a trip to Medjugorje but knew a trip like that was definitely out of the question. No way could I ever go out of the country by myself, let alone fly that length of time. I had a terrible fear of flying and only flew when it was necessary. It was a relief when I reached a destination, but the flights were torture for me emotionally. My knuckles would be white on our arrival.

I had a silly thought that maybe Al would go with me. An hour at church was impossible for him, so why would I think he would go on a pilgrimage? Al wanted us to go to Hawaii, instead. He said spending a week with holy events was not his idea of a vacation.

I couldn't stop reading this book. Every spare moment was spent on the couch reading it. The emptiness and loss of not having more to read left me feeling unfulfilled. I couldn't believe this uncontrollable yearning to learn more.

I talked to the girls at work about Medjugorje every chance I had. A fellow worker in the warehouse was in the National Guard and had just returned from there. People crowded around him to hear his stories, but I had no spare time to join them.

After weeks of not having more to read about on Medjugorje, Leona and I decided to go back to the shrine. I wanted to understand the visionaries' inner feelings seeing Our Lady. *How blessed the six children were to be called.* I wondered how many people in this world were not even aware of this event. I'm sure there were ones who knew and were ignoring, or even laughing at it.

I rushed to the book section again and found *"Medjugorje the Mission"* by the same author. This time I also picked up a video named *The Mother of God Comes to Medjugorje. How could I be so lucky to find this? Now I can feel like I'm there in heart and spirit to witness the sights.*

I couldn't drive home fast enough. I thought shopping for clothes was wonderful, but here I was grasping onto something religious with more gratification than material things. I had purposely left the first book on the end table in the living room by Al's recliner. I hoped it would tempt him enough to read it.

One evening, he stunned me after saying he was already in the process of reading it. I didn't want to make anything of it, and prayed he would want to go with me.

After a short time of reading, I casually said to Al, "Imagine being on the same spot where the Blessed Mother is actually appearing to the children. I can't even comprehend it."

He just took his normal deep breath and said, "I would have absolutely no interest in making a trip like that."

His reply broke my heart. I hoped he would at least think about it.

I read the second book with the same degree of anticipation. I held onto every word Wayne Weible wrote. I experienced the same sadness and emptiness when I finished it. I couldn't understand why this event was taking over every waking moment of my life. I never had a book do this to me. It was an occurrence happening in another country and should have been just an incident to read about...not jump on a plane and go to it. The thought of traveling over there was so strong but I knew it would only happen if Al went with me. If not, it would be left as a dream and I felt foolish thinking about it so often.

When our favorite television shows were on, I couldn't concentrate on them. I would sit and daydream about climbing to the top of Cross Mountain and imagined walking around the location and seeing everything. You would think I was going to be quizzed on the event. If I had such enthusiasm with my studies in high school, my grades would have soared.

Al didn't have the slightest interest in seeing the video I bought. The weekend came and I put it on while he was involved with the yard work outside. I had no intention of moving from my spot until it ended. The film started out by showing a priest named Father Joe Whalen, who led the pilgrimage to Medjugorje along with a tour guide, Charlie Toye, of Reading, Massachusetts.

I listened closely as the visionaries spoke about Heaven, Purgatory and Hell. It was both frightening and captivating at the same time. The visionaries, Vicka and Jakov, talked for a half hour about Our Lady taking them physically to these three locations. I tried to imagine what they had witnessed.

I was learning about all these apparitions and wanted to stand on top of a mountain and scream to everyone this was going on in our world. I wanted them to feel the same excitement that I was feeling. So much crime goes on in this world and people are turning away from God. I couldn't understand why the priests at Mass were not talking about Medjugorje. It was not ever mentioned on television or in the newspapers to reach people. I had to stop and think, *Alberta, you were away from it for years yourself!*

Two books and a video were completed and I still sat each night with a lost feeling. Nothing I accomplished seemed like fun or had any importance to me. My interest in television was gone. *Why is this so important to me? A book is a book. Why is this one getting deeper and deeper inside my brain?*

Chapter 28
Meeting Arlene Albert

I took one more trip to the shrine with Leona to see if something else could be found to bring me peace of mind. I only wanted material on Medjugorje. When I reached the book section, I saw another woman searching the same area. She was a very attractive blonde, in her early sixties, and dressed in a stylish long, tan trench coat. We caught each other's eye and introduced ourselves. She had a friendly smile, was soft spoken, and seemed very out going. There was an instant connection when we talked.

She introduced herself as Arlene Albert from West Warwick, Rhode Island. She was looking for books on Medjugorje herself, so I mentioned the two I had just finished reading. By now I felt like an expert on these apparitions and wanted to help her. Not long into our conversation, I realized she knew more about this than I did. I asked if she ever took a trip to Medjugorje. When she said yes, my heart skipped just to think I was in the presence of someone who had actually been there.

My excitement was beyond words. I knew Arlene could give me some insight into Medjugorje. I got pulled into her story when she described miracles that had happened to other pilgrims, the peace in the village, the apparitions, and the miracle of the sun.

She offered Leona and me a medal which she had bought during her trip. It was of the Blessed Mother and the six children at her feet. Having such a gift filled our eyes with tears. Just knowing they came from Medjugorje was a blessing all its own. Leona had hoped to travel there someday with me.

Arlene asked if we would both like to go with her the following year in May. I thanked her, but explained my fear of flying never mind going such a distance. She promised to keep in touch with me. We exchanged telephone numbers and addresses.

Twenty minutes before, we were strangers and now I felt an incredible desire to know more about her. I never really believed she would call me. How many times do we follow through calling someone after taking their telephone number?

Surprisingly, Arlene and I kept our word and called each other now and then. I told Al about her offer to go on the trip. He looked at me and said, "Go, if you want. It's something you have been talking about for a long time."

I asked him if he would go with me. He had no intentions of changing his mind. I had his approval now and felt completely on my own. I had to be crazy to even think about going on a trip out of the country—not only without Al, but with a complete stranger. It was only August of 1997, and May was long way off. There was no need to give an answer to her now.

With each phone call from Arlene, she would describe, in detail, the village blessed by Our Lady. The information would cause so much passion in me. My emotions were filled with a combination of wanting to be there and trying to fight the terror of flying. *Is it going to be possible for me to do this?* Whether I was at work, home or doing errands, my mind was only on this trip. *Why am I being so immature about making a decision? What's pulling at my heart to go there after reading about it?*

My heart wanted it, but my mind was racing with everything that could go wrong. I started to see how I feared doing thing alone. Here was a woman who seemed nice and our conversations were very relaxed. We talked for hours on the telephone. *Why would I travel with someone I didn't know? What if we did not enjoy each other's company?* I had to stop these negative thoughts. This would not only be the first time I traveled out of the country, but alone.

New Years Day was now upon me and a decision would have to be made soon. A deposit was due to reserve a seat. One night, while talking to Arlene, she said the tour guide was Charlie Toye out of Reading, while Father Joe Whalen would be our spiritual guide.

My mind was blown in realizing that these were the two people in my video. *What were the chances of this happening? Was this a sign from God to go?*

I had to let go of the fear that was over taking me and let Arlene know my decision on the trip. Saying yes gave me fright beyond words. With my history of palpitations and trying to make a decision to go on this trip, my heart was beating like crazy.

The next time Arlene called, I explained my fear of having problems with my fibrillation being away from my doctor and in a strange country. She was very understanding and told me one of her sisters had the same heart problem. We discussed the different medicines and techniques her sister used to combat her problem. Nothing seemed to shake Arlene. She never pushed me or got upset if I changed my mind- which was constant with each phone call. She was loaded with patience.

The next day, I spent my lunch hour away from work and went to the Taunton Post Office to get my passport—just in case. I had had the necessary pictures taken at the AAA office in Raynham the week before, so I took them with me. I started the ball rolling for the trip but was still not sure about going. The idea of flying was pushed to the back of my mind. If I didn't think about it, I wouldn't have to deal with it, for the moment.

Everyone at the office was happy for me, yet shocked I was going to a war-zone for my vacation. After all, the co-worker with the National Guard had no choice, but I did. It was an everyday topic at work and I was surprised they weren't sick of hearing about it. In fact, it did the opposite. My friends were thrilled to be sharing in the details of this event with me.

When they saw I was serious about my decision, they were eager for me to go. My friends were taking turns bringing my Medjugorje video home to see for themselves what was going on there and to learn about the apparitions. The whole office was involved in my plans for the trip, whether they were Catholic or not.

When the itinerary arrived, I made copies to pass out to the individuals who requested it. People were posting it on their bulletin boards so they could follow my daily activities when the time came. They wanted to share the whole trip with me from beginning to end.

I volunteered to take petitions from any co-worker, who wanted their written prayers prayed over, by a priest, or visionary in Medjugorje. They would be presented to Our Lady for her to answer the prayer requests. I guaranteed each person that the envelopes would not be opened. Debbi Bettencourt, our Human Resource Administrator, was back within the half-hour and placed hers on my desk. I collected over forty-two petitions to take with me.

Chapter 29
Roadblocks with Health Problems

Testing my faith—but mostly my desire—to go to Medjugorje, roadblocks were about to hit me the likes of which no one would ever have imagined. Poor Charlie, our tour guide, didn't know what I was going to do. First I was going, and then days later, he would get a call from me saying I couldn't bring myself to go.

Charlie took the time to explain we would be flying on an airbus out of Logan Airport in Boston. He took seven trips to Medjugorje on the plane and insisted they were the smoothest flights he had ever taken. Charlie warned me not to take the flight out of TF Green Airport in Providence, R.I. to Newark, New Jersey. It would be a small prop plane and the flight could be very rough. He advised me to meet the group in Boston.

Finally, embarrassed by my delay in answering, I told Charlie to book me and sent him my deposit.

About four months before the trip, my doctor scheduled me for a colonoscopy test. I had finished the final preparations for the morning procedure, and started to relax in our bedroom for the night. Al was downstairs watching television around 9:00 pm. My stomach was growling from hunger and I just wanted to go to sleep to make the morning come faster. I couldn't wait to eat a full meal the next day.

When my eyes started to get heavy, I leaned over on my left side and stretched my right hand to reach the light on the night stand to shut it off. My heart started to thump hard with a severely irregular heartbeat. It was bouncing like a ping-pong ball, going in every direction at a tremendous high rate of speed. I tried not to panic. For years, I had fought fibrillation, but this was extremely different. It terrified me. There was no pain, but breathing was difficult.

I got myself up into a sitting position and sat with my legs dangling over the bed. Most of the time, changing positions during a palpitation episode would help my heart go back into a normal rhythm. It was not working. I held my hand over my heart and took slow, short steps to reach the top of the stairs. Any excursion during these episodes only made my heart race faster. I called out to Al and immediately he knew by the tone of my voice that there was something seriously wrong. Once he reached the top step and saw me, he tried to calm me. He could see I was short of breath and pale. Al had helped me through many attacks but started to worry himself when they were not subsiding.

I grabbed one of my tranquilizers prescribed for this problem. My cardiologist was in Taunton, forty minutes away, and with any heart problem I knew an ambulance would take me to the nearest hospital, which would be Tobey Hospital in Wareham. That meant I would have a different doctor.

I waited a little longer, hoping my heart would get back into a normal rhythm. After a few minutes, I realized this could be serious. I told Al to call the ambulance. This was something I'd never had to do. My fibrillation could ordinarily be controlled, but couldn't this time.

Al feared leaving me to make the call, but I assured him I'd be okay. I sat again on the edge of the bed, holding my chest and tried to fill my lungs with air. My breathing was shallow and my heart was still racing out of control.

The ambulance department was stationed only a few blocks away, so it was at our door in minutes. One of the three E.M.T.'s ran up to my bedroom. He sat on the edge of the bed and fitted an oxygen mask on me.

The other two E.M.T.'s came up the stairs with a special seat to transport me back down to a stretcher at the bottom of the landing. One of them told Al, "This kind of problem frequently happens when a person is relaxed in bed for the night."

I felt my heart slowing down and returning back to normal once the oxygen was administered to me. E.M.T.'s don't have the authority to determine how serious a person's situation is, so they had to follow through and take me straight to the hospital. Upon my arrival, the emergency department had Dr. Morrow, the doctor on call, examine me. The doctor decided it was best to keep me overnight to make sure they were not missing anything serious.

While I was waiting in the hallway to get a room, the doctor came back to see me. He asked if I had other symptoms that bothered me. I informed him I had been experiencing pain between my shoulders blades for a few weeks and asked if it could be a gallbladder problem.

He said it had nothing to do with the heart problem and would go away. He was not a cardiologist, but he set a follow-up appointment for me to see him when I got out. Once I started to feel better, I was regretting calling the ambulance. Through the years, I handled my smaller episodes by resting and waiting for them to disappear. This was the first time being hospitalized from them.

The administration from the hospital assigned a cardiologist for me. My overnight stay became a week. The doctor ordered a stress test even though my symptoms didn't return. When the results came back showing no serious heart problems, the doctor talked to me and Al before letting me to go home.

The doctor discharged me, but decided to take my heart pills off me, claiming he didn't think they were necessary. I had been taking them for over ten years. The fibrillation started up again and continued every day for a week. I decided on my own to go back on them after notifying my primary cardiologist. It took five days for the pills to get back into my system and relieve the problem.

After having such a serious fibrillation attack, I started to think twice about going on my trip to Medjugorje. It was coming up soon and my fears about going were stronger than ever. *What would I do in a foreign country, an hour away from the nearest hospital? What if they don't understand English and I went into fibrillation again?* By this time, I was a complete wreck. I was sorry I had agreed to the foolish trip.

I called Charlie and told him about my hospital stay and once again, I was having doubts about going. He said a solid decision had to be made within days, especially with eight people waiting to go if I canceled. He told me once he filled my spot, I couldn't retract my decision.

Charlie added to my fear of flying by casually mentioning the trip would involve three flight changes to get there. My heart sank and my knees grew weak just talking to him about it and I had not even left yet. If Al would come with me, my fears would be gone. *How could I be so insecure on my own?* I was really questioning why I ever agreed to go. I was giving up a vacation to Hawaii with Al to travel to a war zone with someone I didn't even know. *Whatever possessed me to decide something so far out of character for me?*

I kept my scheduled appointment with Dr. Morrow, even though I had no idea why I was returning to him in the first place. He asked me how I was feeling and again, I talked about the pain between my shoulder blades and the indigestion in my chest. He looked irritated when I kept talking about it and insisted I was fine. I didn't need any further problems before my trip, so I decided to let it go. Maybe subconsciously, I was wishing for things to go wrong so the trip could be canceled.

I told Al that night I was thinking about canceling the trip.

He looked up from his newspaper, completely surprised, "Really. Why? I thought you wanted to go."

With the way he asked the question and looking so disappointed in me, it made me realize it would be a mistake if I backed out. It was the first time in months I had felt he really wanted me to go. He never talked about it. I had many reasons to go and one was to fill Dad's wish before he died.

Arlene must have been sent from heaven, because she always seemed to call when I had a crisis with my decision in going. I explained about going to the hospital and what had happened.

She said, "You do realize that this is the devil working on you? It's normal to hear about people with serious health problems before a pilgrimage. He's testing you; it's his way of stopping you from completing the trip."

Every waking moment, my thoughts revolved only around the trip. The compulsion to go was mixed with the belief it was necessary. It was like someone was calling me, constantly pulling at emotions.

One morning, I was in bed sick. I was totally overcome by changing my mind every other day. It actually had made me sick inside. The fibrillation occurrence had just doubled my fear of getting these attacks while I was there.

I got on my knees on top of my bed, with my hands up to God and prayed as hard as anyone could. My frustration had me actually screaming out loud, "Please, God, help me with this. I can't handle this decision. If it's the devil working on me, let me defeat him."

I asked St. Michael to drive Satan away and get my mind healthy for this trip. I prayed to St. Raphael for healing of my heart problems and asked for peace with my decision. I wanted to stick with going and let it go. I actually broke down and cried from the feeling of being lost and weak because of a decision to go somewhere. *Why can't I back out? No one was making me go.*

All my friends at work were excited waiting for me to take this trip. Each day my office was filled with people chatting with me about what I was going to experience. There was so much faith restored in some employees and I knew they would lose it if I didn't complete the trip. All my talk about God, Our Lady, miracles and a little town in Bosnia would be lost forever for them.

Maryanne Stevens, who was in customer service, gave me a petition from a friend of hers. The friend's son, Todd, was in his early twenties and had brain cancer. He was dying and the doctors said he would probably not live another month. His mother put a lock of Todd's hair in an envelope. Friends with cancer were hanging onto the hope their petitions would be blessed with a cure. People who wished to travel there themselves were living their dreams in my future experiences.

I knew something, or someone, was pulling me to Medjugorje. This was not my decision. All I knew was this had to happen—even though I did not know why.

Arlene called and explained Our Lady calls each individual herself to this location. "If you don't go, Our Lady will be disappointed." This made me understand why the desire to go was so strong inside of me: I was being called.

It was down to five weeks before the trip and I had a doctor's appointment with my cardiologist. We discussed what symptoms caused me to be rushed by ambulance to the emergency room. He told me to push my fears aside and not to stop myself from living because of one bad experience. If another attack came, he advised me to quietly lie down somewhere and take a pill. "If it doesn't go away in an hour, take another pill and just rest." He did tell me not to get overtired because that can bring on fibrillation.

With the doctor's appointments behind me, I put everything in God's hands to get me there. My comfort with the decision had one more test. The pain I complained about between my shoulder blades? It got worse. The emergency doctor had told me to ignore it. Here it was four weeks before the trip, and poor, Al was taking me to another specialist to get the symptoms checked. The surgeon confirmed it was my gallbladder and recommended me having surgery to remove it right away. This way, I would be fit for the trip. Recovery time was a month. He scheduled the pre-op testing the next day, and surgery in two days.

I had no time to really think about it.

He saw the shock on my face and asked, "Do you want to go on this trip and have a serious gallbladder attack? Get this over with so you can go with no worries."

The surgery was completed with no complications and I had two weeks to heal completely. Our Lady must have really wanted me in Medjugorje. The only thing I didn't question by now was the fact I *had* to go. I knew deep down that if this trip was not taken, I'd probably never go. Once fear is faced head on, it's not so intense; it's thinking about it that gives you doubt.

Chapter 30
Flight to Newark International Airport

It was now May twenty-fifth, three days before my trip, and the excitement of it all was coming together. The night before, Al surprised me by making a fabulous lobster dinner for the two of us. A chef would have had a challenge beating Al's homemade scallop dressing. Candles placed on the table and a bottle of wine added to the exceptional meal. It was such a special and loving thing for him to do for me before I left. He was not one for romantic words, but his actions always said it all.

On Saturday, May twenty-eighth, the moment had come to leave on my trip. It was a combination of anticipation and nervousness. I wished Arlene had met me at Logan Airport in Boston, but living in West Warwick, Rhode Island, only made sense for her to fly from T.F. Green Airport in Providence. She was boarding a prop plane to meet the group in New Jersey. The jet sound much better to me. As much as I feared flying, I wanted to hear and feel the power of a jet engine under me, when we took off.

The thought of leaving Leona behind was heartbreaking. She claimed the lumberyard was too busy for her to take a week off. She never flew and feared it worse than me, if that was possible. I had strong feelings she could not overcome the fright and that was the real reason she stayed home. It was something I could understand. We both had planned and prayed to share this trip together. Before I left, she gave me her rosary beads and Dad's cross pendant to take for a blessing in Medjugorje.

Al drove to Logan Airport. I had hoped someone in my area was going on the same trip so we could have shared in the expense of a van and save Al the long trip. I kept wishing he was coming with me, but finally accepted the fact that this journey was mine, not his.

We arrived at 11:00 am at the airport and Al parked the car in front of the terminal to check-in my luggage. My only wish now was to find the tour group. I longed to see anything or anybody familiar.

I had no idea where to go in the airport and followed Al like a puppy. No matter what direction he took, he had me on his heels. Al had always made decisions about traveling, so I depended on him to get me to the right gate for my flight. It had never crossed my mind that someday I might travel without him.

Charlie had mailed a package out to everyone. It contained a red baseball cap to wear so we would all be identified as Charlie's Angels from The Spirit of Medjugorje Tours. No one from the group was waiting in sight when we reached the gate. I was trying not to push the anxiety button inside me. Since he left the car unattended, Al could not stay much longer. I tried to hide my fear from him.

Al waited ten minutes to see if someone from the group would show up. If just one person from the group would have arrived, it would have put me at ease.

It finally reached a point where Al had no choice but to leave. He gave me a hug before departing and I smiled, waving like a frequent traveler before he turned the corner. While my insides were in knots, I faked being relaxed. I honestly wanted to grab onto my husband's ankle when he headed back to the car. This was either going to make me or break me.

It was twenty minutes before the scheduled flight was due to leave, and I was still standing alone. *Where was the group?* My doubts had me thinking this might be the wrong area. Countless times I checked my ticket to see if it was the correct gate and airline. If it wasn't, I would have been in tears not knowing what to do or where to go. Except for one woman sitting in a corner, the gate area was completely empty. I couldn't believe a flight was ready to leave with no people waiting to board. *I have to be in the wrong place,* I thought.

Having had time on my hands, started me thinking nothing but negative thoughts. Maybe I *was* nuts traveling to a country with a war going on. What if our flight hit turbulence or worse, crashed? I went up to a sales counter to get a magazine to read and purchased hard candies in case my ears popped during the flight. I had to keep moving. The more I pictured myself going on the plane, the sicker I became.

Ten minutes before boarding, a group of fifteen to twenty people walked up to the gate. It seemed like an eternity before they arrived. They all had red hats! What a tremendous relief, seeing Father Whalen and Charlie Toye. I recognized them both after I had seen them in my video at home.

I was going to be completely alone on the flight, not knowing one person traveling to Newark, N.J. I went over to Charlie and introduced myself. I thought he might not be excited meeting the insane woman he had been speaking to for the past five months. To make my first impression with him worse, he told me they had been waiting at the baggage area for *me* to arrive. I had over-looked the itinerary page that stated where to meet.

It was now 2:00 pm and we were called to board our plane. Although it felt like my legs didn't belong to me, they were moving. My heart was racing. On the outside, I looked calm, but I felt like a two-year-old in a strange place.

I imagined my legs straight as boards and someone pushing me from behind to get me on the airplane. *How can a person have so much paralyzing fear?* I didn't want an attack of fibrillation from anxiety. I prayed over and over again, to help me stay relaxed.

The group was divided and sat in different sections of the plane. Not one person on the tour was near me. I noted where everyone sat, so when they got off the plane, I would see what direction they headed next. I sat myself at the assigned window seat, when a young girl in her late twenties sat next to me. She casually admitted in her conversation that she had fear of flying. I knew she was not going to be giving me any support if I needed any. We spoke to compose ourselves from nerves.

The take-off was smooth. As we ascended, I held my breath and dug my fingers into the armrest until we leveled off. The weather could not have been more perfect. There wasn't a cloud in the sky and the sun was shining. The Lord gave me my first gift.

A combination of excitement and peace came over me. As I looked out the window, I mentally spoke to Our Lady. *I'm coming home to you. We have stepped over the devil and beat all the roadblocks with heart problems, surgery and fear.*

The plane hit some small turbulence, but I remembered what my friend, Heidi, from work said to do when it happened. "If there is turbulence, close your eyes and pretend you're in a car on a bumpy road." Believe it or not, it worked. If anyone watched me, they would have wondered why I was smiling from ear to ear. I was so proud of myself. Nothing else mattered in my life at this moment, not even my family.

This was the first time I was doing something by myself and for myself. Of course, I almost had a breakdown, but I was here. The flight was going to be forty-five minutes before we landed in Newark, New Jersey. I sat back and looked out the window, and wondered what I was going to experience on this pilgrimage.

Chapter 31
Reunion with Arlene

We landed at 3:00 pm in Newark, N.J. I blended right in with the group, running to keep up. Independence was trying hard to kick in. I looked at my tickets and tried to learn gate and flight numbers. The first thing I wanted was to spot Arlene so there would be a familiar face. It would be the first time seeing her after our one meeting at LaSalette Shrine seven months earlier.

On our way to the boarding gate, I finally located her. Arlene laughed when she admitted almost not recognizing me. That was not too reassuring to me at the time. We all headed for the assigned gate for our next flight to Prague.

Arlene began describing the flight on the prop plane and how bumpy it was the whole trip. She said, "Lucky you didn't take off from Providence."

She was right about being lucky; I would've had knees like jelly getting on the next flight.

It was amazing, as I watched everyone grouping together from all different states. Some mingled and talked with former friends who had made other pilgrimages before to Medjugorje. Introductions were being made to complete strangers with such ease.

I listened as individuals spoke about being at Medjugorje. I was shocked hearing how many trips others had made, and wondered how anyone would want to do the same thing every year. *Wouldn't they want to have some fun at a vacation spot sometime? After all, how many of these trips could they take without being bored?* I couldn't imagine leaving Al home every year while I went on trips alone.

I immediately felt relationships begin to form among the group. I was astonished to witness this automatic closeness with everyone. Usually, when Al and I traveled, no one took the time to even smile at us.

Arlene introduced me to a very good friend of hers from Warwick, R.I. His name was Eddie Sousa and he had his son, Ed, Jr., with him. Ed, Jr. was studying to become a priest and this was also his first trip to Medjugorje. Little did I know the tight bond that would also develop with Eddie.

I would soon learn how spiritual renewals work on these trips. I didn't feel this, so it was hard to understand it. My goals were to deliver all the petitions from family and friends and to make the trip for my father.

Chapter 32
Flight to Prague

Before boarding the plane at 5:30 pm, Father Joe blessed the group with holy water and prayed for a safe trip. I thought, *I'm now experiencing what it is like to be on a pilgrimage.* Passengers not on the tour watched with curiosity.

We entered the airbus, which held over four hundred passengers. Arlene and I shared two seats together by a window. I was happy with the seating arrangement, because I never liked being squished in the long middle row.

Arlene and I were locked in together for a full eight hours while we flew to Prague. To my complete astonishment, there was never any time of uneasiness. The only thing we found missing was time to catch our breath from talking non-stop which has never changed through the years.

With the ease between us, it felt like we had known each other our whole lives. As each hour passed, we learned about one another's likes and dislikes. Our Lady certainly knew who to pick to transport me to Medjugorje.

We talked for hours about everything from our childhood years right up to the present moment. Her last name was Albert, and I had a twin brother, Albert. We both had sisters named Leona. One sister had heart problems, like me, and we both had a brother that died. There were six children in my family, and Arlene had fourteen. Our interests blended together, but the most important conversations consisted of Medjugorje. I couldn't hear enough about it.

Time past fast because of our constant talking, and before we knew it, it was eleven o'clock in the evening. I tried leaning my head back to rest, and maybe even get some sleep, but the excitement had me too keyed up. I remembered the doctor had advised me not to get overtired, but could feel it happening. Knowing that we would be in Medjugorje the next day brought my anticipation higher.

When midnight arrived, we passed through the time change and the dark evening sky was changed into a beautiful sunrise. I never had this experience while traveling. I sat and watched the sun shine through the windows.

The bright sun's reflection off the plane's wing hurt my eyes, and I turned away. Arlene stared directly into it smiling with contentment. She never blinked once.

Eddie walked down the aisle and leaned over me, and asked Arlene if she saw the miracle of the sun. Both of them shared this great phenomenon. Arlene described the sun spinning with soft shades of pink, blue, purple and gold. She said when the colors encircling the sun, it pulsated.

"Can you see it?" she asked.

The brightness was so powerful that I couldn't imagine how anyone could look directly into it. It was blinding. I took fast, short glances, and my eyes watered. I feared they could be damaged by staring at it. I leaned back letting the two of them enjoy their blessings. I knew in time, Our Lady would show me if that was her wish.

Chapter 33
A Day at Prague

It was 7:45 am when we landed in Prague. Charlie was right about the smooth ride of the airbus. It felt like we had been sitting in a living room the whole way. We did not hit turbulence the entire eight hours. It would have been a great experience for Leona's first time flying.

We came off the plane exhausted from the long flight. We carried small overnight bags for our stay in Prague. Our luggage was transported to another plane for the next day air travel. What a relief that we did not have to drag our baggage anywhere when we were so tired.

The bus from the airport took about a half-hour to get to the Kladno Hotel. It had a strange appearance because it was built not only tall, but very narrow. It didn't look like our hotels in the United States, but I expected this.

The elevator was old and it could only carry two people at a time. During the war, it was used to carry only food carts. They had never replaced it with a modern one. But at this point, the atmosphere didn't matter to me. All I wanted was a bed and shower.

Charlie gave us two hours to wash and get refreshed. We were scheduled to meet the group in the restaurant for lunch before a city tour. Between the time change and no sleep since I left the house, my body felt like it weighed a ton. *Please God, don't let me get my fibrillation.*

Arlene and I tried to rest for an hour, but not even a snooze was possible. I started to feel weak and nauseated from lack of sleep. We both decided to get up and go meet the group. The restaurant was small, with nice decorative paintings and colorful potted flowers. It was relaxing to get the chance to know everyone.

After lunch, the bus was waiting to take us to the center of Prague. When we reached our destination, Charlie explained where to meet and what time to the ones who wanted to go their own way. It was a good decision to leave my pocketbook at home and bring my backpack. It left my hands free; a feather by now would've been too heavy to carry.

The artwork on the buildings was breathtaking. It's said that Prague is one of the most beautiful cities in the world and the sights proved it. I loved the cobblestone streets. The details on each building made me wonder why our old historical buildings back home are ever demolished and rebuilt for modern ones. The older they are, the more splendid they seem to be.

Charlie pointed out the important sights and talked about their history as we walked through the city.

Father Whalen scheduled a Mass at 2:30 pm at Our Lady of Victory Church where the Statue of Prague was located. When Charlie opened the door, all I saw was gold throughout the whole church. There was so much gold in the statues, lights, and the décor that it caused me to just stand there in amazement after entering.

We entered through a side door that led to a gift store where I purchased the Prague and Holy Spirit medals to save especially for the men back home. I took fifteen of them, hoping that would be enough.

I walked into the church and went up to the altar to see the Statue of Prague. It could've been easy to miss. The statue itself was not only gold, but the whole alter wall, right up to the ceiling, was gold. It was hidden from view. I could not believe I was kneeling and praying in front of this famous statue of Jesus. So much history resonated all around me.

My prayers centered on Todd, who was fighting for his life with cancer. A boy I had never met before, but his presence was deep in my soul. He was due to pass away before my return. I prayed for God to let him live at least to give him more time. I held the envelope that contained the locket of his hair along with all the petitions. I laid them down at the altar rail. There, I prayed for each individual who needed healing.

Father Whalen called us to sit in the pews while he started a Mass in this holy church. He prayed over all the letters we had brought from home and blessed them through the Holy Spirit. When he mentioned praying for the people who could not come, I thought of Leona. She would've loved witnessing all this with me. I told her before leaving that the Blessed Mother must not have been calling her at this time. With all my roadblocks before leaving on this trip, I had developed the knowledge that nothing on Earth will get in one's way if Our Lady is calling you.

I held my friend Rita's rosary in my hand as Mass was being said. I took turns holding different rosaries given to me, including my father's.

After leaving the church, we continued our walk and came upon a long, low bridge. The whole length of it was filled with artists painting and selling their pictures. European artwork was something I had never seen back home. There was a peaceful joy in watching the artist painting portraits in person.

During our travels we saw old churches, quaint little restaurants and wonderful statues in and outside of every building. Except for attending Mass, we walked from 1:00 pm to 7:20 pm non-stop. By now, I had severe pain in my legs and hips. I honestly did not know if I could make it to the bus. What a welcome sight to see it waiting for us at the corner.

There were so many things to do and see throughout the tour that not many in the group stopped to eat in the restaurants. People craved the cold drinks more from the hot weather and long walk. The bus dropped us back at the hotel and a late supper was served for the group. Arlene and I couldn't wait to go straight to bed. My mind was in a daze and my body begged for sleep. There was little conversation with Arlene that night and sleep was thankfully not a problem.

Chapter 34
Split

The next morning, we were up at 5:00 am to get the 7:20 am flight to Zagreb, the capital of Bosnia. What a difference in alertness, after getting a full night's sleep. It was going to be easier to face another full day of activities without being exhausted.

The bus met the group in front of the hotel and took us straight to the airport. Once we got to the terminal, we settled in our seats to wait for the arrival of our plane. An hour later, it taxied down the runway. People were now picking up their overnight bags and headed for a side door.

I expected to see a jet and instead, a prop plane was facing me on the runway. The flight had been a little bumpy, but to avoid being on edge, I concentrated only on the enthusiasm of knowing today we would be in Medjugorje.

When we landed in Zagreb, we had one last air travel to the city of Split. There was a forty minutes wait before we left. At 1:20 pm, our plane departed and a new world was about to open for me traveling to Bosnia.

The airport in Split was very small. It didn't take long to get our luggage. We went out the front doors to board the motor coach. About ten buses were lined-up in the parking lot waiting to take the tourists to their destinations. It was a three-hour ride to Medjugorje.

Arlene was excited to be back for the second time. She tried to remember which side of bus she sat at last time to view the Adriatic Sea. She said it was spectacular. Here was a poor country, destroyed by a war, and Our Lady chose to appear in this devastated land.

I studied the homes as we traveled through the countryside. There was very little conversation between Arlene and myself. I sat by the window and was content in the silence.

It was summertime now during our visit to this country. The view with the cattle and sheep roaming the open fields, had given me a feeling of stillness.

Children stood by the roadside, watching the buses pass by. As we looked back at them, they waved and smiled. Their clothes were very simple and plain, and it had me thinking about my clothes at home. They are packed so tightly together in my closet that I have trouble pulling them out. *Why do we need so much?*

I started to think about how much money I paid for this trip. Here were families that had probably never left home. So many will die never having seen the other side of the world, but will still be happy knowing God gave them so much. I believed their pleasures came from their family life, tending the animals, and working in the fields. I analyzed each sight as we traveled. I wondered how many people standing along the roadside had lost family members because of the war.

The bus driver slowed almost to a stop when he came to a cemetery on our right. He told us that only soldiers from the war were buried there. The caskets were all encased above the ground.

As the bus regained speed and bounced on the unpaved roadways, I was amazed at how much was seen out my window in a short span of time. It would've been gratifying to talk to the residents and listen to their stories.

This was not a vacation trip where a person is entertained, eating gourmet meals or sitting on a beach enjoying the ocean breeze. *What brings pilgrims back year after year to this little village after seeing it once?* A half-hour into our trip and I could feel my heart being touched.

Half way to Medjugorje we stopped at a replica shrine of Our Lady of Lourdes, built by the bishop of Split, after he visited the original at Lourdes, France. The bishop of Split realized that he had in his diocese an exact replica of the cave in France. This shrine is an active healing site with the same spiritual and healing charismas as the original. The statue of the Our Lady of Lourdes is encased in a grotto that faced us as we stepped off the bus. The area had rows of open benches so people could pray. Groups of nuns were walking around everywhere. Charlie told us they lived at the monastery right up the hill and came down to pray here daily.

Father Whalen prepared to say Mass outside at the grotto. I was sure it would be a refreshing experience to attend Mass outside. People who passed by sat on the benches to join in the service. When Mass was completed, we made a short visit to a tiny gift store.

After a half an hour, everyone boarded the bus and settled into their assigned seats. We were excited about getting closer to Medjugorje, and Arlene and I started up our conversation again. Father Whalen led us through one decade of the rosary and everyone blended in with the prayer. If I had not learned the rosary during Dad's illness, I wouldn't have had the chance to say it with the group.

When we finished praying, I looked out of the window to take in the majestic mountains.

Arlene leaned over with a warm smile and whispered, "So, how do you feel, being in Medjugorje?" My emotions hit me and tears started down my checks. I looked back out the window to keep from breaking down completely. Arlene saw me fighting for control and didn't press me to talk.

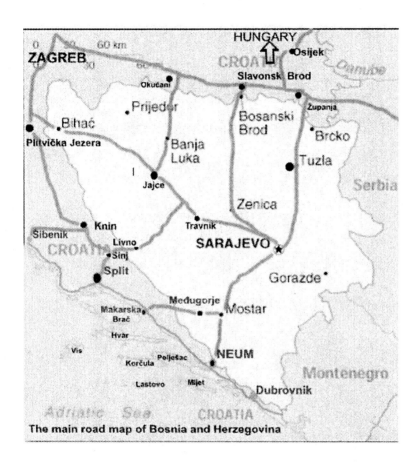

Map of Medjugorje

Chapter 35
Arrival at Medjugorje

Then it came into view...M*edjugorje.* The bus moved very slowly on the narrow dirt roads. No big resorts or hotels were visible. The private, stone homes were very close to one another. Contrary to what I expected, the village was not crowded.

From the right side of the bus, Cross Mountain faced me. Of the things I wanted to accomplish on my tour, one was climbing to the top. It was so far off, yet, it stood out so magnificently. To me, this was not any ordinary mountain; miracles happened there everyday. The huge cross placed on the very top was the famous landmark where so many miracles were said to have happened.

I tried to grasp the reality of being here. Months ago, I never expected the chance to share in this event. Every word I read in my Medjugorje books stayed in my heart, mind, and soul. It seemed so far out of reach to me back then. I had made it, and my feet were about to step onto holy ground.

I had no interest in watching what the group was doing around me. My eyes searched for the familiar locations seen in my video. Little did I know when Albert showed the tape of the visionaries at my parents' home in East Falmouth, that I would actually come to Medjugorje. I would've laughed at the mention of it.

The bus came to a stop in front of a three-story home where we were going to stay for the full week. It was owned by a woman named Nada and her son Neven Cililc, who were our host. To our right was a large group of pilgrims entering St. James Church. No matter where one stood, its tall steeple stood out. The village was small and it seemed like most things would be within walking distance to us. Only a few passing cars traveled on the road. Taxis were parked and lined up along the main street to take pilgrims wherever they wanted to go.

We stood outside the bus as the suitcases were stacked up on the ground for each owner to claim. Charlie started to call out the names and the numbers of our assigned rooms on the second floor.

Debbie and Lori had bought me a new suitcase for Christmas to take on my trip. It was the largest in the group. The suitcase required two men to carry it up to my room because of its weight. It never occurred to me while packing that elevators wouldn't be available. The two men were relieved that the bag didn't have to leave my room until my departure.

The bedroom Arlene and I shared was very comfortable. It contained three single beds, a bathroom, a closet, blankets and towels. The families that owned homes opened them up to pilgrims. This was a wish Our Lady asked of them. Clothes would be washed if they were left outside your door. Two homemade meals each day were prepared, with fresh vegetables from their gardens.

The bathroom had a shower that had a cement base floor. The shower curtain was held by a large, circular ring. Water for the showers was only available in the morning and only between certain hours. It was impossible for their water supply to handle the amount of people who come to Medjugorje.

Arlene and I used the middle bed between us as a drop off for our belongings. As we placed our items in our designated areas, we could hear laughter and conversation from the others getting settled in their own rooms. Sounds echoed as the suitcases bounced on the steps as they were pulled up to the third floor, above us. Father Joe was in the next bedroom and we both worried he was not going to get much sleep surrounded by so many talkative women.

The excitement of the up-coming events could be felt. Our arrival erased the fatigue we were all feeling. Resting was not in anyone's thoughts once we unpacked. I suddenly felt a connection to everyone after the short time traveling with the group.

Once our room was organized, Arlene was anxious to become my private tour guide and show me the area. It was late that afternoon and we were on our own. We didn't have to come back for supper. If one didn't want to eat back at the house, there were restaurants in the village. People could stay with the group, or go their own way the whole trip. Charlie had scheduled a tour the next morning with a couple of the visionaries.

Medjugorje was a small village and it could be traveled in twenty minutes by taxi. The main street had vendors that were lined up one after another. Except for special statues or pictures, each one sold the same religious items. The gift shops were the ones that had the special displays.

Since there was a whole week ahead of us, I didn't want to start buying articles right away. The important things were mainly the visionaries, church events, Mass, Confession, Cross Mountain, Apparition Hill, Blue Cross, and prayer. The visionaries stressed the best gift you can bring home to anyone were the rosaries.

We started our activities by heading straight to St. James Church. It was incredible to see the multitude of people gathered around it. People from all over the world were either entering or exiting the huge church. It was a constant flow. If our churches or Adoration Chapels back home were filled like this, we would be living in a different world.

I had heard that each Mass was so packed sometimes you couldn't find a seat inside. Speakers were placed around the church so the people sitting on the benches outdoors could hear the priest give the services. Mass was celebrated every day at between 7:00 am and 11:00 pm. They were said in different languages like Croatian, French, German, Italian, English and more for the millions of pilgrims. The doors closed at twelve midnight and Arlene said the people still didn't want to leave the church.

We sat on a bench outside and watched the people walking around the church. A Mass was being said in Croatian. What a beautiful language.

My eyes took in the magnificent church, the same one pictured throughout my book. It was the famous place where Father Jozo protected the six visionaries when the police were chasing them. The persecution of the visionaries, their parents, relatives, the parishioners, priests, and even of the pilgrims began immediately after the beginning of the apparitions. The visionaries were taken for police investigations and psychiatric examinations, but it was always stated that they were healthy. The same conclusion brought about further examinations done in the following years.

Father Jozo, pastor of Medjugorje at that time, was arrested on August 17, 1981, two months after the apparitions, and sentenced to prison by a Communist court to three and a half years of hard labor. He had endured 18 months of horrendous torture and had been released on the condition that he never returns to St. James Church as a pastor.

St. James Church is the *Heart and Soul of Medjugorje*. Our churches back home should make us feel the same as this holy one. I remember when ushers were needed to help people find seats in church because so many attended. Not today. We see so many elderly, but where are the young children who should be filling our spots when we pass away?

Next to the church was a gift shop that carried hundreds of books and articles. Many were written by Father Slavko Barbaric, and I couldn't wait to hear him speak to us. I bought *Follow Me With Your Heart* by Father Slavko in case there was quiet time to read.

After we purchased our books, we walked again to St. James Church to sit and people-watch. There were at least ten or more confessional enclosures outside the church and each had large lines waiting so people could find peace in their hearts. Each one had a sign above the door, showing which language the priest spoke.

Everyone who stepped out from the confessional boxes seemed to radiate serenity. Others walked out with red eyes, probably from crying after having a weight lifted from their soul and being given a new life.

Our first night at Medjugorje fell on Pentecost Sunday. As the darkness settled in, the cross on Cross Mountain could be seen all aglow, like red coal. Witnesses have said if you climbed to the top to see this event, the cross would appear normal and not appear lit or glowing.

At the end of the evening, a few of us from the tour group congregated at Viktor's Restaurant. It was located four houses down from where we stayed. We treated ourselves to ice cream sundaes and it became our ritual each night during our whole stay.

Evening became a special time for me. There was so much peacefulness in this village. Certain sounds of Medjugorje became embedded in my mind. Our bedroom faced the street and when I lay in bed, everything became so still I could hear the sound of tires passing over the stones in the dirt road. Very few cars traveled by and when they did, each one could be heard. The groups, who returned late to their assigned homes, would kick up pebbles with their shoes as they walked. Their voices became whispers of private conversations under my window. The atmosphere gave me such a rush of tranquility and it sent me into a deep, relaxing sleep each night.

Medjugorje was not just a place of sounds. It filled my very soul spiritually when I saw people during the day walking with their rosaries, praying, attending Mass at St. James Church, or sharing Adoration with Fr. Slavko. People with flashlights, at night, could be seen going up Cross Mountain. My whole day was a time of learning, feeling, talking and hearing prayer. I never felt like something was missing from my life being in this village. If anything, it *gave* me life.

Strangers talked openly about why they had made the trip to Medjugorje. Jeff Gallagher was one of them. Arlene and I met him while eating at Viktor's Restaurant the first night. He decided to tell us his story as we headed back to our house.

He was a handsome, tall, slender man in his late thirties wearing a close-shaved brown beard and mustache. Jeff had had the same excitement coming to Medjugorje as each one of us when we were called by Our Lady. Just a month before his scheduled date to leave on the trip, Jeff had an accident while driving his company truck. He developed severe neck injuries and the doctors didn't know if he would ever be able to walk again.

He looked at us and said, "I'm really not supposed to be here."

Jeff started to describe what had happened to him the night before when he decided to climb up Cross Mountain. He was going up by himself with a flashlight and wanted to give thanks to Jesus for healing him and allowing him to make the trip.

He offered up his sins by making the climb barefooted with the discomfort and pain endured. Every step consisted of hitting rocks that were wet, slippery, sharp or jagged. There were no clear pathways for walking to the top. The people in the village have always kept the paths as nature developed them. Pilgrims have descended countless times with their feet bleeding.

Jeff continued telling us when he was halfway up the mountain, a miracle happened. The joy on his face could be seen as he spoke. Jeff described hearing a crowd all around him yelling, cheering and condemning Jesus to be crucified. He was given the power to hear not only the rocks being thrown at Jesus, but the cursing against Him. Every individual voice could be heard. Jeff had no doubt that God gave him the power to hear the people who had actually condemned Him to His Crucifixion.

I asked if it frightened him and he remarked, "For some reason, it didn't. I just kept asking Jesus over and over again to forgive me for my sins as I continued up the mountain." Certain people are chosen by Our Lady and Jesus to witness something beyond our world. This was Jeff's time. He said that experience would help him the rest of his life to trust in the power from Heaven.

We stopped a few moments in front of our house and thanked Jeff for his story. Arlene and I said goodnight to him close to midnight. You could see the contentment he had after sharing the blessed event with us. He waved and went off in another direction. We never saw him again during our stay, but he was someone who touched my life. He was another person, like me, who had faced and combated roadblocks before his trip.

I never wanted the night to end. I had no desire to sleep. If it was possible to exist without it, I would have omitted it completely. Back home evenings were filled with rushing to do errands and fighting traffic after work. The day ended watching television and going to bed around 9:00 pm. I did not take the time to find a quiet corner to pray.

After spending less than twenty-four hours in Medjugorje, I could sense a change in myself. Having time to be alone and completely separated from both my family and my routine had showed me that I became closer to God being in a quiet place with no distractions.

As we settled in our room, our beds started to look appealing. When the lights went out, we suddenly had energy again and acted like teenagers. Here I was, feeling like I was at a pajama party in my younger days. Complete foolishness had us in tears from laughter. I couldn't remember the last time I laughed so much that my stomach ached.

I started to observe the pleasure I had with being myself with Arlene. It made me see that Al and I had taken everything in our lives too serious. We didn't find humor in our mistakes or in the way we did silly things. I now learned that taking things lightly in life, and bringing more laughter in my day, could heal a heart from hurt or take pressure off making decisions.

Chapter 36
St. James Church

I woke to the same sounds that had engulfed me when I had gone to sleep. People were already up and heading to wherever they had to be for the morning. Not once did I ever hear someone yelling or horns blowing from the few cars that did pass through the village. I looked over to my left side to see if Arlene had awakened. She was doing the same: just listening to the sounds of Medjugorje.

Taking showers was a challenge for us. The curtain enclosure would never stay up for some reason. We had to sit on the base of the shower floor, trying to keep the water from going over the bottom rim. We just joked about it instead of bothering anyone in the household. It was offered up as a sacrifice.

As we walked down to the dining area, the group could be heard, blending in with the morning conversations. There were no special seating arrangements, so everyone could mix in with different people during each sitting. This gave us an opportunity to get to know new people each day.

Father Whalen started each meal with a blessing over the food placed on the tables. Breakfast was not fancy, but it had all the necessities. Our Lady asks us to fast each Wednesday and Friday only with bread and water, so bread was the main entrée for those who gave up a big meal during their stay. Fasting on those days was something I couldn't do, or maybe I didn't try hard enough.

Different toppings, consisting of butter and jellies, were available to go along with the assorted homemade breads. Fresh oranges, strawberries, apples and bananas were placed in large bowls. Sometimes hard-boiled eggs were served. I was never disappointed, or had the need to search for more. Coffee, a variety of juices and water were the only drinks. Soda was never placed on the tables, but was available in vending machines outside. I found it odd for modern vending machines to be in Medjugorje but maybe there was a large request from pilgrims.

Our mornings started with the 10:00 am English Mass at St. James Church. The front entrance and the two side doors already had an eager crowd lined-up and waiting. The Croatian Mass was just ending. It didn't take long for new pilgrims to learn that the seats at the service were taken within minutes once the doors opened.

In 1897, St. James Church was as a small place of worship. From 1936-1966, construction of the church was delayed due to WWI, WWII, and Yugoslavia's civil strife. Finally, in January 19, 1969, the church was blessed even though the interiors were not finished. The people wondered why such a large structure was necessary for this small village. The answer came after June 24, 1981, when Our Lady appeared to the six visionaries. Once the event spread around the world, and large groups of pilgrims started to come to Medjugorje, the villagers understood it was a plan from God. Now, to their amazement, it had become too small.

Arlene told me to grab any seat available when the doors opened. She said, "If you hesitate for a second, every seat will be gone. We may not be able to sit together so we'll meet outside after Mass."

All three doors opened and people were trying to get in at the same time the crowd was trying to exit. The procedure was in a controlled manner without anyone yelling or being rough. I had no choice but to follow the person in front of me because people were pushing forward from the back of the line.

I spotted Arlene on the left getting into a pew up front. We were separated and I was suddenly fighting to find an open seat. I fought panic that was trying to overtake me. People were coming from every direction and rushed to fill any free section. It seemed the church was packed in seconds, not minutes.

I had to grab any seat near me before they were all taken. A couple followed right behind and pushed me further in the pew. People were shoulder to shoulder leaving no room to place any belongings on the seat.

I started to feel like a sardine, and took a deep breath to control the sensation of being squeezed in an enclosed section. The steps at the foot of the altar and the center and side aisles were thick with the crowds standing. They swallowed up any open area in the church. Tiny canvas folding seats were positioned at the end of the pews. Pilgrims spilled out the doors and others sat on the outside benches to listen to the Mass from the speakers around the church. I never saw anything like it in my life.

Within minutes, thirty to forty priests in red and white garments approached the altar. The sight was so colorful and soul-moving, my eyes filled. It was difficult to keep from sobbing. Seeing so many priests from all around the world, in one location, adoring Jesus made my heart come alive. True inner love was in the atmosphere and an instant connection came from every person in all directions. We were all there for one reason; to adore our Heavenly Father.

There was not a moment I wanted to study people to see how they dressed or acted. My eyes were glued to the altar. The presence of Jesus and Mary was so powerful that it could be felt within me. Experiencing this emotion made me imagine how the visionaries' must feel seeing, hearing and talking to Our Lady. No wonder they say there are not words on earth to describe it. I was so blessed to be called here to become a part of this holy service. To think this movement had been going on everyday since 1981, it floored me. All these years I had ignored this event.

Mass started and I relaxed, watching the sights on the altar. After the gospel was read, another priest began telling his own life story about how and why he wanted to be ordained. With each Mass a new priest would do the same. Not one was embarrassed to talk openly about the bad things they did before making the changes to turn back to God and serve Him.

During the service, the words to the songs had me wanting to break down again. Hundreds were singing so loudly the church vibrated from their voices. Holy Communion was served by priests at the altar, down each aisle, in the back of the church, and seven priests even walked outside to present it to the people on the benches.

It made me sad to think how empty our churches are at home. I thought, *Where are God's people?* How lucky we are He is beyond judging us for our human faults. He waits through the years, lovingly and patiently, with open arms, for us to return. Many people spend their life trying to find the right path leading to Him. He forgives every sin, fault and weakness, even when we commit the same mistakes over and over again. Forgiveness is a gift He gave us with His death.

Arlene and I met in front of St. James Church when Mass ended. I couldn't believe that I managed to sit for over an hour in church. I walked out feeling the Holy Spirit. Never before had a Mass touched me so deeply.

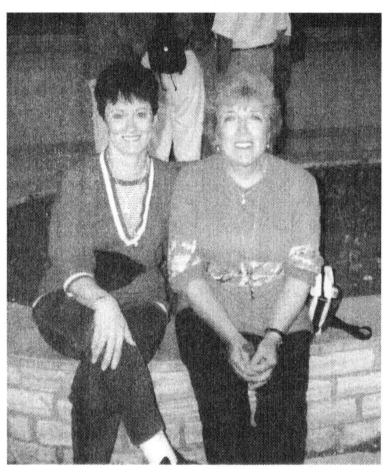

Left: Alberta & Arlene

Chapter 37
Visionary Mirjana Dragicevic

After Mass, we met our group at a small chapel in back of the St. James Church. This was one location where the visionaries had had their early apparitions. We waited for our tour guide, Draga Ivankovic, who is a cousin to four of the visionaries and a recognized authority on the events of Medjugorje. *How do I explain the wonder of meeting the person you read about in a book?* There she stood right next to me. She, like the others, wanted no fame, but it came anyway after the books and articles were written about the events. She does not see the Blessed Mother, but devotes her life speaking to anyone who comes to Medjugorje. Our Lady's apparitions are repeated to millions of pilgrims each day.

It's remarkable how the visionaries continue to speak to pilgrims every single day. It's done faithfully because they are truly devoted to the Blessed Mother. The visionaries are just as human as we are: they get sick and have bad days, too. They give up their lives to lead us to the endless happiness with Jesus and Our Lady. It must be a heavy burden for them to keep the secrets from us.

Before the tour got on its way, Draga explained it would be impossible for her to join us at certain locations. She was in her third month of pregnancy with her first child and couldn't exert herself too much by climbing or taking long walks. The first visionary on our itinerary was Mirjana Dragicevic. The route of travel to her home was on a pathway through a thinly wooded area, which led to an open field.

The region started to remind me of when I was a small child living in West Springfield, Massachusetts. As a young child, I investigated trails in the woods behind our house and they never seemed to end. The sounds of nature from the squirrels, birds, and running brooks would come upon us as we pushed deeper into the forest, leaving our rural neighborhood behind. Walking with the tour group made me reminisce about my childhood fun and pleasures. The same smells from wild flowers and tall grass were coming back to me.

It brought me back to a time I had forgotten. I remembered how Albert and Leona shared in these adventures with me. We pulled long, thin grass out of the ground and placed it between our two fingers to blow through it. It gave a whistle sound. The three of us carried pails to catch frogs in the streams on our way. Each trip challenged us on who would find something amazing to bring home to show our parents. They were special memories.

We passed two elderly women who labored in the open grape fields, wearing veils and black dresses. I expected young girls or only men to be doing this strenuous work. They made it look like second nature working in the heat.

Cross Mountain was far in the distance on our right. The field on the left was covered, as far as the eye could see, with over-grown, red poppy flowers. They swayed in the light warm breeze as if they were dancing to music. I was tempted, with my youthful heart, to run and fall in the middle of them.

As we came through the end of the woods, the path continued between stone houses. The yards were bursting with the most enormous and brilliant red and yellow colored rose bushes. I had never seen roses so large. I figured the hot climate in Medjugorje must have been the reason they looked so healthy. Roses are Our Lady's favorite flower and I'm sure the villagers are very aware of it.

We finally reached the home of Mirjana and joined others pilgrims that had already congregated in front of her house. It was not long when she came out and approached the white, wooden fence that surrounded her property.

Her interpreter explained to us, in English, that Mirjana was not feeling well. She had the flu and was running a fever. What a strain to be under and yet she had the strength and love to talk to the crowd. Through it all, she found the energy to give us a smile.

Mirjana Dragicevic-Soldo was born March 18,1965 in Sarajevo. She is the second oldest of the six visionaries. On June 24, 1981, she was the second one to see the Blessed Mother appear that day. Her family lived in Sarajevo and she spent summers with her grandmother who lived in Bijakovici.

She had had daily apparitions from June 24, 1981 till December 25, 1982. On this last date, Mirjana received her 10th and final secret from Our Lady. Mirjana was the first seer to receive all ten secrets. Our Lady told her with the last apparition that for the rest of her life she would have one yearly apparition on March 18th. All the visionaries, who have received their ten secrets, have a yearly apparition with Our Lady.

Starting August 2, 1987, on the 2nd day of each month, she hears Our Lady's voice. The prayer intention that Our Lady confided to her is: **for unbelievers…those who have not come to know the Love of God.**

Mirjana is married to Marko Soldo, who she has known since they were children. They have two children. She meets with the pilgrims daily when they visit Medjugorje. She also has helped at the orphanage in Medjugorje since the war.

When Mirjana started to speak to the group, she stated, "So many priests have lost their way. In Medjugorje we always show respect for our priests. Never speak ill of them…pray for them. If you're not comfortable at a church, find one that you like and worship there."

Mirjana continued, "Our Lady has told us that if you have a choice between coming to see me or going to church…choose Mass. There, you receive my Son and He is truly present on the altar."

Mirjana wanted us to understand the importance of being in the presence of Jesus and receiving Him. She stated further, "Our Lady wants everyone to pray the rosary and it's not enough to simply pray.

It's not enough to just quickly say some prayers, so that one can say they prayed and did their duty. What she wants is for us to pray from the depth of our souls and to converse with God."

Speaking in a soft voice she said, "Our Blessed Mother wants us to pray more and we should love God as our Father. We should accept the messages of prayer, fasting, conversion, and reconciliation that God is sending to the world through the Blessed Mother of Jesus. If we do this, we'll not be afraid of anything no matter what the future may hold."

Each of the six visionaries are receiving ten secrets from Our Lady. When the last visionary receives all ten, they'll give them to the chosen priest, ten days before they happen. The priest will read them to the world, three days before they are to occur.

The secrets are written on a cloth that can't be destroyed even by fire. The priest, in turn, will not be able to read them without the help of Our Lady. The secrets will be read one at a time, depending on the dates. They'll name the place, dates, time, even minutes where they'll occur. These secrets contain major events that will happen to the world. That's why it's important to convert now.

When Mirjana completed the talk, she bent her head down in prayer. We stood silently as she prayed for all of us. Once she finished, she smiled and turned to walk back into her home. The group broke up to go separate ways since the rest of the morning was our own time.

Chapter 38
Oasis of Peace/Apparition Hill

Arlene wanted to show me the Oasis of Peace Chapel that was just around the corner. The shrine was off the dirt road and the entrance had a long, winding, cement walkway bordered with white and pink roses with yellow honeysuckle on each side of the path. The small chapel was hidden within a forest.

There was a sign outside the area asking for silence upon entering the chapel. When the two heavy wooden doors were opened, it revealed how small and empty the chapel was, with only two people inside kneeling in prayer.

There were only roughly ten rows of pews on each side of the center aisle. The old, uneven wooden floors creaked as we walked. The noise echoed all around us from the stillness. I started to walk down to the front row.

In the far left corner was a statue of the Crucifixion of Jesus. It was built to the actual height and size of a man. It had hair on His head and legs instead of just a solid porcelain statue. Blood was upon Him everywhere, even at the bottom of the statue, to show his excruciating suffering. Deep open cuts and bruises were embedded all over His body in detail. The crown of thorns showed the severe and bloody injuries caused by the wounds in His forehead and scalp.

I could see the reality of His agony. I fell upon my knees. He's truly the King and Savior of all men. My eyes filled up and tears rolled down my face. Anyone with compassion would be affected by this sight. For the first time in my life, I visualized the actual pain He must have endured as I looked up at Him. No human could have stood such torture for our sins. Jesus gave up His life for us.

I found myself asking God to forgive all of us for what we did to His only beloved Son, Jesus Christ, and Our Savoir. Our sins of fear, jealousy, anger, lust, greed, and hatred killed Him. The only person on Earth who loved us unconditionally was taken and hung like a criminal. I couldn't turn my eyes away from His torn body hanging on the cross. I studied every inch of the statue from head to toe. I only saw a man. We forget this. He was a human being like us all. What a gift we had tossed aside.

I wanted to package the statue up and deliver it to every single church, so everyone could kneel adoring Him. They could gaze upon Him and see the reality of who He was and what He did for us.

How weak we are as humans needing to see to believe. The Bible, which is the greatest book of faith, is tossed aside by many. It's the life story of Jesus told by his chosen disciples, who not only walked on this Earth with Him, but ate and slept with Him. It's the Church teaching that God is Infinite. *"He was, He is and He always will be" (Ps 90:1-2).*

After leaving the chapel, our souls were so full of peace that we walked in silence. Our next stop was straight up the road to Apparition Hill. This was where Our Lady first appeared to the visionaries.

As we came to the bottom of the hill, hundreds of pilgrims were already in a procession going up following Father Slavco. I only became aware of the climb facing me. It was probably nothing to others, but not for me. Any climbing, especially stairs, can bring on fibrillation faster than anything else.

The hill was not gradual in its ascent, but started straight up from the street. There were rocks and clay three-quarters of the way up before a grassy knoll could be reached. This was going to be a trial for me. I didn't want to let Arlene know it was going to bother me.

I was wearing light weight, tan summer slacks, sneakers and a red, cotton three-quarter sleeve shirt. The clothing was already too heavy for the weather and the climb was only going to add to my body heat. I was already perspiring. Having my backpack over my shoulders at least left my hands free to balance myself as we started the climb.

I spotted a cross, high above the crowd that was being carried up Apparition Hill as hundreds of pilgrims followed. As each station was reached, a new person would carry it. We joined in the rosary that was already in progress after merging into the crowd. People from all over the world were saying the prayer in many different languages all at once. It was beautiful the way our voices blended together. You could feel the love for Jesus and Mary from every stranger reciting it.

I was ecstatic knowing we were going to the actual site where Our Lady first appeared to the children. It wasn't easy seeing beyond the crowd in front of me to judge how far it was to the top, and it was all uphill.

The path was very narrow when we finally reached the brush. It was thick with wild rosebushes. As I brushed by them, the thorns clung and grabbed onto my summer slacks. The hill leveled out into a more open area when we reached the peak. It was a relief to be able to walk straight.

The crowd was starting to kneel around the cross that had been placed where Our Blessed Mother had first appeared. It was erected high upon a mound of rocks and placed on the highest point of the mountain. The peak was elevated so high above the landscape below that the view was breathtaking. The warm breeze had a cooling effect on me, to some degree.

The whole village of Medjugorje was spread out beneath us. The view from the mountain showed the land divided into sections with the open fields and plowed farmland. St. James's steeple stood so high above the homes, it made it easy to spot the church.

Arlene was already praying on her knees at the foot of the cross when I came upon the spot. The sun was hitting the steel cross directly, causing it to sparkle. It stood tall to mark the location where the visionaries first saw her.

I tried to imagine the event. *Right where I'm standing, it happened.*

My heart leaped with both excitement and the greatest feeling of affection. The visionaries had stated that they had seen Our Lady coming down from Heaven holding baby Jesus in her arms, and I tried to visualize it.

My emotions were no different from what everyone was experiencing near me. All of us had the same call to come to this village. The trip was a gift for each person to feel, standing at this divine spot. Our Lady blesses each person and only asks us to pray and do whatever the visionaries are relaying to us.

Pilgrims had started to departed from the mountain. Arlene and I sat and talked about our spiritual feelings before leaving. What a renewal this was for me.

After an hour, we started to slowly descend from the hill. At the bottom was a small, enclosed booth where a vendor was selling food and drinks. Both of us ordered something cold to drink to refresh ourselves. The young girl serving us said the weather was extremely hot for this time of year. The temperature was already in the nineties. Little did we know it was going to get even hotter.

Chapter 39
The Village of Medjugorje

On our way back, we passed through some gift stores in the village. My eye caught an outstanding statue of the Blessed Mother on the floor. Her detailed features and the soft colors on it, made it so beautiful. I mentioned to Arlene how it would be fantastic to buy it because it was so different. I thought of having it shipped home.

Giving me a hesitant look, she replied, "Wait till you get home. I have a strong feeling that Al is going to buy you one while you're here."

Laughing under my breath I remarked, "Al, buying me a statue? I don't think so, Arlene!" She hadn't met him and I felt she didn't know his personality. Yet her remark made me hold off in case a miracle did happen.

Little time was spent shopping, due to the heat and the fact we had to walk to the other side of the village to get to our house. Our excursion back was very peaceful traveling towards the open fields again.

On our way, Arlene and I wandered through a back trail. We came upon a family dwelling that was constructed right at the edge of the path. Their living quarter was only a hut containing open gaps between the sideboards, which allowed us to see right through the home. I couldn't help but wonder what the family did in the cold winter months.

Behind it was a fallen down structure, something we would consider to be a barn. It was very low and rickety, with a crumpled roof that was not intact. Three sides of the building were barely standing and it leaned halfway to the ground. One side had already collapsed. It gave no shelter whatsoever for the animals.

An elderly man and his wife were feeding their goats and anyone could easily see that they owned nothing. The property contained only the two worn-out buildings. There had been no rain since we were there, and it left the path in front of their property with dry, cracked mud after the hot sun beat down on the top soil.

The couple gazed at the both of us with warm smiles as we passed by. They probably wondered about us the same as we did them. I thought of how many pilgrims must pass in front of their property day after day, yet they showed no signs of being annoyed. At that moment, I longed to speak their language so I could learn about their lives and to understand them.

The animal's surrounding area gave off an extremely foul and unpleasant odor due to the sun hitting their stables and the heat intensified their scent. I held my breath as we passed by the area. We were careful to avoid stepping in the animal waste.

The hot air didn't give us any relief when we reached the open fields. The full sun was beating down on us. It drained the little energy I had left from the day. The soft wind made the tall blades of grass sway together in slow motion. The sounds of June bugs could be heard but not be seen.

Along the way, vendors had tents set up on the paths to protect them from the sun while they sold their items. Blankets were laid out on the grass displaying homemade afghans and holy items to catch the eye of the passing pilgrims. We bought rosaries because the prices were cheaper than at the stores in the center of town.

Arlene and I finally came upon the field that was bursting with poppy flowers. There were African men and women standing among the overflowing flowers taking pictures. Arlene asked if they wanted her to take pictures of them and they could do the same for us in return.

They started to speak French and Arlene impressed me when she mixed right in and started to speak it fluently. I knew she was French and born in Maine but did not know she spoke the language. We took turns snapping pictures and then continued toward our village.

It wasn't long before we came upon a shaded but thickly wooded area. I couldn't get over the number of birds singing in the trees. No matter where we traveled, the noise from the continuous flocking birds was overpowering. We were surrounded by them. It was enjoyable to hear their sounds because I've always felt flowers and birds were the most beautiful things God created.

When we reached the village, people could be seen wandering through the small market places looking for the best deals. On Sundays, the really devout Catholic vendors would close their gift stands. They give up the profit to spend the day worshipping.

Arlene and I wanted to rest our feet after walking all morning. We went to the benches at the statue of Our Lady in front of St. James Church. The statue was built from the visionaries' descriptions to a sculptor on how she appeared during the apparitions.

The statue is carved and painted all in white with Our Blessed Mother standing on a cloud. She is said to never touch the earth when she appears. Her long veil came down her back to the bottom of her gown. She is shown as a young girl, in her twenties. Our Lady's right hand is placed on her heart and the left is held up. The statue is placed on a cement block with bright pink roses growing in a circular area below her feet, surrounded by a large, black wrought iron fence.

Each visionary sees Our Lady the same. They have already several times declared that it is impossible to describe in full detail how the "Queen of Peace" looks. Her beauty surpasses our every attempt. Their explanation has been, "Her beauty can't be described—it's not our kind of beauty—that's something ethereal -something heavenly— something that we'll only see in Paradise—and then only to a certain degree."

Her physical description: 5 feet, 5 inches, she is slender, around 132 pounds, from eighteen to twenty years old, a long, oval, face, her eyes a wonderful clearly blue, and black hair. They once asked Our Lady how she was so beautiful and she remark, "Because I have love in my heart always."

We sat on one of the benches to pray. I became aware that Arlene was looking directly at the sun wearing her sunglasses. She asked if I wanted to see the miracle of the sun. I could tell she desperately wanted me to share in her gift.

Each time I looked up, the sun was still blinding. It was impossible for me. I repeated again, "If Our Lady wants me to see it, she'll show me." I didn't want to seek out occurrences that happened to others. I took comfort in knowing that if it was meant to be, miracles would be placed in my path.

Eddie Sousa spotted us and came to join in our conversation. I had not seen him since the bus had dropped us off at the house. He had accompanied his son, Ed Jr., and they had gone in a completely different direction with another group. He started to watch the sun turning colors along with Arlene.

This was the second trip to Medjugorje for both of them. I would be leaving at the end of the week and they had made arrangements to stay another week longer. They were retired and had the time. I tried not to think of returning and leaving them behind.

Eddie startled me with an unexpected question. "Well, Alberta, how does it feel to be at Medjugorje?"

My emotions surfaced again and I broke down in loud, long sobs. I couldn't control myself.

He sat next to me and put his arm around my shoulder. "It's very emotional, isn't it? I did the same thing the first three days when I arrived here last year."

Eddie started to tell me about his years as a police officer for the West Warwick Police Department. He was irrelevant and initially he'd had no interest in the spiritual world or life. He explained how his wife, Donna, had been to Medjugorje a few times and kept asking him to go with her. He didn't mind her taking the trips, but he had absolutely no desire to go. It reminded me of Al's way of thinking. For some unknown reason, Eddie suddenly had no other longing but to come to Medjugorje. Like all who are called, he read everything about it. Now, here he was on his second pilgrimage, with his son.

Ed, Jr., was studying to become a priest but was struggling with his doubts about whether or not this was really his mission. He was told by others to visit Patrick and Nancy Latta when he came to Medjugorje. Nancy was an interpreter for Father Jozo and had helped many priests with their vocation. Ed, Jr. was now praying for some sign to help him make a decision.

Chapter 40
Visionary Ivan Dragicevic

Charlie had scheduled the group to meet another visionary, Ivan Dragicevic, that afternoon. Ivan was going to tell his story in the village park, and like all the visionaries, he would have an interpreter. We arrived at the park around 2:00 pm and a huge crowd had already gathered. The location was shadowed by trees, so the heat was bearable. The temperature was climbing and anything that helped keep us cool was a break.

Ivan is the oldest of the male visionaries and was born on May 25th, 1965 in Bijakovici. Our Lady had been appearing to him every day since June 24, 1981. She had confided nine secrets to him. Ivan was married and resided in Medjugorje with his family. His wife was a former Massachusetts beauty queen and they both live in Boston some months out of the year. He was asked by Our Lady to: **pray for the young and for priests.**

Ivan arrived and started by saying, "The apparitions have made a big difference in my life. I've arranged to make praying time during the day. Before, my life had no meaning. Now, I'm filled with inner contentment. The first time I saw Our Lady, a change occurred in my soul and in my heart. I often avoided prayer, but now the difference is so great I really can't describe it. I'm not sorry Our Lady revealed my future. I'm confident and not afraid, because I know who leads me and therefore, I'm not afraid of death. All people should feel that way."

Someone asked if he was ever aware of people around him when Our Blessed Mother appeared to him. Ivan replied, "I'm in total ecstasy and never aware of anything or anyone around me. My total concentration is only on Our Lady." Ivan spoke for about a half an hour and by then, the heat had become uncomfortable, so he ended it, after answering a few questions.

Chapter 41
Miracle of the Sun and Birds

After listening to Ivan talk, Arlene and I went back to Our Lady's statue. Arlene was now determined for me to witness the miracle of the sun. She picked up my sunglasses and handed them to me. "Put these on and do what I tell you. Look up for a second and then look away. Keep doing this till you don't have to turn away from it," she stated.

I tried to please her by doing as she instructed. I did this four times. Gradually, each interval didn't seem as intense as the time before.

Finally, I could stare right into it and not turn away. A host covered the front of the sun except for the circumference. Pilgrims, who come to Medjugorje, describe the host as the same shape as the one received in Holy Communion during Mass. The colors of blue, green, red and pink were forming around the rim of the sun. Our Lady had let me see the miracle! Here I was, looking right into it without my eyes watering. *How could this be?* Multiple colors all blended together with the same result as a rainbow. We both sat together sharing this great miracle.

It was around 5:00 pm when we started back to the house because supper was ready to be served. The table we chose was right next to the kitchen and each family member could be seen working together. I watched closely as each person had certain responsibilities with preparing the meal so it would be served all at once hot and on time. I couldn't imagine cleaning up twice a day after thirty people or more at each sitting.

Pitchers, containing water and juice, were already placed on the table for us to help ourselves. The cold juice went down nicely after a day in the hot sun. I'm not normally the type to drink a lot of fluid, but with the intense heat, I craved cold liquids. During the day, many people were seen carrying bottled water with them everywhere. This was something I didn't do, either, but probably should have.

After the meal, we sat awhile and conversed. There was excitement in the air when someone told their stories about what they saw and did on the trip. I soon discovered why friendships would never be lost once you shared the experience of a pilgrimage with strangers.

It was a beautiful night, so we decided to go back to St. James Church to sit on the benches. It was nearly 6:40 pm, the time when Our Lady appears to Vicka, Ivan and Jakov. She will appear to them, even if the visionaries are out of the country.

As we waited, the loud sounds of chirping birds above caught my interest. I looked up and saw them flying back and forth in every direction around the nests they had built under the eaves of the church.

I suddenly remembered my book had mentioned the birds stopped all sound and movement when Our Lady appears. This was an event I wanted to personally witness. As they came and went with food for their babies in the nest, my eyes never left them. There were hundreds of them flying. I was surprised that none of them were colliding with the speed of their flight and with so many in the air.

Exactly at 6:40 pm, the priest inside the church could be heard on the outside speakers telling everyone that Our Lady was appearing. Every Mass stops at this time. At that precise moment, every activity from the birds stopped. There was no movement at all. They were nowhere in sight. The apparition lasted around seven minutes. Once it ended, the birds went right back into their routine as though nothing had happened. It was something one has to see with one's own eyes. Even the creatures had felt her presence.

After the event, we chattered awhile with friends we had met during the evening, and then went back to the house. I was exhausted and decided to relax and go to bed at a decent hour. It was already close to ten o'clock. Arlene went downstairs to the front patio to join the others so she could give me some quiet time to sleep

Chapter 42
Picture Embedded in Rosary Pouch

The next morning, Arlene informed me that Pat and Nancy Latta had unexpectedly stopped by the house to explain to our tour group how they both came to Medjugorje to live. They had talked about how their lives had changed. I was heartbroken to have missed their story.

Following breakfast, Arlene took me to the post office, which was situated at the other end of the village. I wanted to call Al to let him know we arrived safely. This was the only place public telephones were available for outside calls. It was early and the shops were not open.

Our direction of travel led away from the busy section of the village. Everything was motionless at 8:00 am and no one seemed to be stirring. It was enjoyable walking in the early morning, cool air, instead of experiencing the heat of midday.

The post office had one room, with a lobby containing six telephones on a wall and one person at a window for services. It felt good to hear Al's voice when we were connected. Talking to him brought me right back to my familiar world, like before my trip. As strange as it may sound, Medjugorje felt like it wasn't connected to the world we live in today.

I love my family, but already longed to stay here. I had started to feel that this way of life in this little village was how it was intended to be for everyone. I dreaded the idea of returning home to my old lifestyle.

It's up to each and everyone one of us to change our ways. Old habits of rushing here and there to accomplish the everyday tasks had me worried my praying would fade into the background.

I was trying to tell Al everything I'd seen and experienced in the past few days. He had to interrupt and give me some terrible news. He told me my ex-sister-in-law, Anita Lopes, has had open-heart surgery. Her husband, Sonny, had a stroke from being upset over her mishap and both were in the same hospital. They own the Lopes Construction Company in Taunton and both my daughters, Debbie and Lori, worked for their aunt and uncle.

I panicked. Sonny previously had two major heart attacks. Being so far away, I began to question how quickly travel arrangements could be made if anything happened to either of them.

Al sensed the distress in my voice and said, "Calm down. The best thing you can do is to pray for them to get better while you're there."

I knew he was right. He always had the right answers. Rosaries are the strongest prayers for the sick. This was a time to turn to faith. I asked him to tell the family we would be praying for them. Arlene knew by my expression that something dreadful had happened to someone. Hearing the details she said there was time to catch the 10:00 am Mass to pray for them.

We headed back and got in the line already forming at the side door of the church. I observed a boy in a wheelchair ahead of me. He looked to be in his early twenties. Judging from his warm smile, he seemed to be in high spirits. One person, out of millions, that was disabled and had come to Medjugorje. They pray for a healing or inner serenity, so they can face each day with their poor health. People from all over the world were coming for a miracle.

His father was adjusting him in the seat to make him more comfortable. I asked what his son's name was and he replied, "Frank." I promised to say a prayer for him and he thanked me. Strangers were passing through my day, leaving me with the desire to help them.

Meanwhile, the number of people that arrived got larger and created a tremendous line outside. It was a miracle in itself to see how hundreds of pilgrims could squeeze into this church. As we waited, Arlene took her rosary beads out of the pouch. My eye caught something gold on the inside. It looked like rust spots. I couldn't imagine why rosaries would leave a rusty spot inside a clean pouch. Arlene noticed it at the same time and kept rubbing it, thinking the color would come out of it. I suggested that she turn it inside out to get a better look at the stain.

Arlene turned the pouch and looked at me with a shocked expression. "Tell me what you see to confirm what's facing me," she said.

There, as clear as day, was the outline of the Blessed Mother from the waist up, with her head bent down, covered with her veil. It was detailed in two different tones of gold. The outline also showed her holding the baby Jesus. He was leaning His back against her and you could see His knees bent up plain as day. It was stained in the lining of her rosary pouch. We studied the rosaries themselves but they were clean, with no rust on them. Arlene stated that last year, the rosary chain links had turned gold.

Before Arlene had the chance to put them away, the church doors suddenly opened. This time, I knew to move in promptly with everyone else so I could get to an unoccupied pew. Arlene and I were fortunate to find a seat together this time. As the Mass began, I started to pray for Frank, Anita, and Sonny. I would later learn that both Anita and Sonny had recuperated. *How strong are prayers with faith?*

There were so many men in church who were not shy to join in with the singing. Their deep voices blended in perfectly with the women's higher-pitched tones. As I looked around the church, I couldn't find one person who was not singing.

I sat and wondered why people back home treat Mass like it's such a chore? On special holy days, like Easter or Christmas, parishioners perform their "yearly duty" and attend. Years ago, I was one of them. No one feels they need God anymore. It's only an hour a week out of our lives. What are we all doing to our souls?

Chapter 43
Confession and Penance

Following the services, we found contentment once again just by sitting on the benches outside the church. My concentration this time was on the confessional boxes and I noticed the priests were already inside. The lines were very small at this hour.

I reflected on how many people today are receiving Holy Communion without going to confession. If they were in fact going, why was my church or others I attended so empty during the confessional hours on Saturdays? It was impossible that every person in church on Sundays who intended to receive had not sinned. I sat feeling ashamed about not going monthly myself as we are asked to do by Our Lady.

Friends have often remarked that we don't have to go to confession anymore. I'm stunned they believe this. It's so wrong. We *do* need to go to confession. It makes us more *aware* of our sins. That's one of the reasons for confession. Otherwise, we all keep sinning and don't take notice of it. The thought of doing wrong doesn't even enter our minds. So many people think they can go straight to God and confess, without a priest. The priest gives us absolution to cleanse our souls and brings us closer to Our Lord. They are the only ones given this right from God. Many Catholics don't realize what a gift this is for us.

The Medjugorje book I read mentioned that visionaries stressed the importance of confession. They were educated about it themselves the first year Our Lady appeared to them. During this time, the Blessed Mother started to allow the crowd to feel her presence. Some claimed they felt heat or a current in the space they were told she was positioned.

After a very short time, she told the visionaries to put an end to individuals touching her. She explained the people were so full of sin, that they were soiling her white gown. The Blessed Mother wanted them to go to confession to cleanse themselves from their sins and to do it as soon as possible.

Ever since I read this, it gave me the insight and knowledge about how strong our sins are against God and our very own souls. We are given many graces and the strength to combat Satan when we ask for forgiveness in confession as well as with our penance. Because we do not see or feel these gifts, we don't even think about their existence. Too many of us have to see to believe. Everything has to be proven. What has happened to faith? The more we pray from the heart, the more Jesus helps us realize this. The Holy Spirit leads us out of temptation. Leaving God out of our lives, leaves us wide open for Satan to control us.

Any disruption in our life is the devil's work. He loves to have marriages fall apart, he causes fighting and yelling, he keeps us weak in faith so we question if God even exists. The farther he keeps us from Our Savior, the more he owns our souls. He relishes anything we do against God. We may lust for sex while dating, living with someone or outside of marriage—that is when Satan is in command and tries to take us away from God.

Our Lady told the visionaries that most souls go to Hell because the number one sin is lust. Society does not even blink an eye with couples not being married involved in sex. I pray to be worthy enough to go to Purgatory before crossing the threshold of Heaven. It's a place of suffering to cleanse our souls from these sins before going to Jesus. We have to be completely pure before we enter the Kingdom of God. At least in Purgatory, you have hope that someday you'll be with God. This is why confession is so important. We have to be as free from sin as we possibly can be.

It's written, *"Be sure of this: if the master of the house had known the hour when the thief was coming, he would not have let his house be broken into. You also must be prepared, for at an hour you do not expect, the Son of Man will come."* *(Luke 12:35-40)*

Thinking about this reality made me decide to get in line myself and make a good confession while I was in Medjugorje. There was an incident that lay very heavy on my soul for years even though it had been confessed in the past. I couldn't shake the guilt feeling deep inside my soul and felt it should be confessed again. Since I was in Medjugorje, it made me feel closer to God. *This is the place for God to really hear me and understand how sorry I am.*

As I went into the English confessional box, I prayed God would lead me to the most sympathetic priest in Medjugorje. I took my time explaining to father what was bothering me. He was very compassionate and understanding. *Thank you, God, for leading me to the most understanding priest. You've answered my prayers.*

Then I made the worst possible move. My confession was almost completed when I admitted this had been confessed to another priest years ago. At that instant, I was sharing a tiny box with the priest having only a drape separating us. He lost all control and got offended beyond words. He replied back in such a loud and irritated voice, it made me jump out of my skin. I was no longer in a spell of holiness.

He firmly stated to me, *"Don't ever confess a sin a second time or carry guilt once you are forgiven. When a priest forgives you...God forgives you. If you carry guilt, you're letting the devil win and control your soul by making you feel God is not loving, compassionate or forgiving. When it's forgiven, it's forgotten in God's eyes!"*

I can't express the degree of intensity in his tone. I never imagined a priest displaying such dissatisfaction with someone in confession. I told him, "I never thought of it as the devil doing this to me." He then gave me my penance.

I opened the small door and walked out of the confessional. I lowered my head, searching only with my eyes, to see if a crowd was waiting to see the person who just upset the priest. I was flabbergasted that people were still in line waiting to see *this* priest. My penance this time made up for the years of carrying my guilt. That priest left an outstanding impact on me forever. I now look at confession and forgiveness as a gift from a loving God. Carrying guilt afterward only weakens our faith. It was the greatest lesson.

I went back to the bench and took out my rosary beads to say my penance. Al had given me these rosaries as an anniversary gift. A few people at work couldn't understand my thrill in receiving them.

One person even replied, "Rosaries for your anniversary? I don't see how that kind of a gift would make you happy."

They missed seeing the meaning of this gift in my heart. My husband didn't go to church, but took the time to look for the right rosary beads for me. He chose them himself. Al had witnessed how much prayer meant to me. His gift gave me hope and faith that he himself was being led to Jesus through conversion.

Cross Mountain faced me as I said my rosaries. The cross on top of it was in the distance, with the morning sun hitting it directly. I'd read that it weighs 15 tons, is 22 feet tall and was built in honor of 1,933 years since the birth of Christ. It has become a symbol of faith, hope, and charity and a means of penance and conversion, first for the villagers of Medjugorje, and now for the multitude of pilgrims who come here. Many pilgrims have alleged to have had apparitions of the Virgin Mary at this site.

The sun sent a warm sensation through me as I prayed. I shut my eyes and leaned back against the bench. Nothing at this moment was as important as the peaceful private corner where I was feeling the presence of Our Lady.

Chapter 44
Visionaries Jakov Colo and Vicka Ivankovic

Arlene and I met with our tour group that was walking to the home of the visionary, Jakov, to hear him speak. Jakov Colo was born on March 6th, 1971, in Sarajevo. He has had daily apparitions since June 25th, 1981. Jakov is married with three children and he lives with his family in Medjugorje. The prayer intention that Our Lady had confided to him is: **for the sick**.

Arriving at his home, Jakov and his interpreter were on his front porch waiting, at the railing for the other group that was approaching. He's the youngest of the six visionaries, and was only ten-years-old when Our Lady had originally appeared.

Jakvo talked about an episode that happened at this youthful period. He and Vicka were taken physically to Heaven, Hell and Purgatory with Our Lady. He was so terrified to know that this was going to occur that he had begged Our Lady to just take Vicka. Both of them witnessed people in Heaven clothed all in white gowns and weaving baskets. Jakov didn't wish to give a description about Hell at all. "There are no words to illustrate the horror of it," he alleged.

Jakov told us that Purgatory was a dark, murky environment where souls suffer while being purified before entering into Heaven. There are three levels. Souls that have severe sins at the time of death start at the lowest, which is closest to Hell for their suffering. People on Earth are the only ones who can pray for them to get out of Purgatory and reach Heaven. He said, "We are to be prepared for our death at all times."

Jakvo continued by saying he and Vicka vanished for over twenty minutes as family members searched the nearby area for them. I was mesmerized, thinking about their experience and the knowledge that was obtained from traveling beyond our life. They have all the answers to the questions we are all asking.

He ended his story and offered to respond to any questions. September 12, 1998 Jakvo received his tenth secret from Our Lady. She told him he would have one yearly apparition on Christmas Day. It was told that he cried for hours from the heartbreak after his last daily apparition with Our Blessed Mother. He would no longer see her on a daily basis.

Jakvo thanked us for coming and prayed over us. The group of pilgrims then turned to walk towards Vicka's home. Vicka Ivankovic-Mijatovic was born on September 3, 1964, in Bijakovici. She still has daily apparitions. Our Lady had entrusted nine secrets to her so far. Vicka wrote about her experiences in the book, Thousand Encounters with the Blessed Virgin Mary in Medjugorje (1985). Vicka lives in Krehin Gradac near Medjugorje. The prayer intention that Our Lady confided to her was: **for the sick.** It's the same request as Jakov's.

The crowd gathered, standing shoulder to shoulder in the backyard, waiting for her to emerge from the house. The flow of people filled every inch of the property. The individuals who couldn't get through the gate, had to listen from the street.

Vicka came out a side door on the second floor onto a small balcony. The steep stairs led down to the courtyard, where she chose to come only halfway down the steps to address the group. If she was at ground level, everyone wouldn't have been able to see her through the crowd. Even still, the multitude of people made it impossible to see her entirely. Now and then, I would get a glimpse of her when someone would change positions. It had been hard getting comfortable standing a long length of time.

Vicka is recognized as the "smiling visionary." She seems to take total delight in talking to every pilgrim who travels to Medjugorje. Hundreds of pilgrims come to see her, hoping to be healed.

As Vicka described her daily apparitions with Our Lady, Arlene leaned over and whispered, "Imagine...her eyes have looked right into the eyes of Our Lady!"

I tried to picture something so sacred.

Vicka stated, "Those who follow the Ten Commandments have nothing to worry about, those who love and care for others have the Holy Spirit, and those who are loyal will be shown ways around the danger that looms."

She continued, "God is giving so much time for these apparitions so that all may come to conversion. Our Lady wants to make certain that all people, from all creeds and beliefs, have this opportunity. She can't help anybody who doesn't want to change, who doesn't come back to God, who doesn't put God first. If you don't do this *now*...it will be too late."

Vicka tried to answer as many questions as she could and then proceeded to pray over all of us. It was ten minutes of silence and Arlene thought it was unusual for her to pray this long with the pilgrims.

The sun was blazing down on us. Being stationed in one position for such a length of time, with no shade, caused a young woman in front of us to almost pass out. A friend supported her while pouring water over her head. Vicka continued with closed eyes another ten minutes before finishing. When people realized she was done and noticed her leaving to go up the stairs, they started pushing from all directions to get a chance to try to make contact with her.

The last two visionaries were not in Medjugorje at this time and we wouldn't be able to meet them. Charlie said it was rare to visit even four out of the six. We weren't fortunate to see the other two visionaries. The fifth visionary is Marija Pavlovic-Lunetti who was born on April 1, 1965, in Bijakovici. She still has daily apparitions. Through her, Our Lady gives her messages to the parish and the world. From March 1, 1984, to January 8, 1987, the message was given every Thursday, and since January 1987, on the 25th of every month. Our Lady has entrusted ten secrets to her. She's married and has three children. With her family, she lives in Italy and in Medjugorje. The prayer intention that Our Lady confided to her was: *for the souls in Purgatory.*

The sixth visionary is Ivanka Ivankovic-Elez. She was born on June 21, 1966, in Bijakovici. She was the first visionary to have seen Our Lady. She had daily apparitions until May 7, 1985. On that day, confiding to her the tenth secret, Our Lady told her for the rest of her life, she would have one yearly apparition on June 25th, the anniversary of the apparitions. Ivanka is married and has three children, and she lives with her family in Medjugorje. The prayer intention that Our Lady confided to her: **was** *for families.*

Chapter 45
Father Slavko Barbaric in Adoration

Before the night's activities took place, we went back to the house to get some rest. While we climbed two flights of stairs to get to our room, I was glad we weren't assigned to the third floor: with the combination of stair climbing and the high temperature every day, it was a miracle my health was holding up. All my torment back home was for nothing.

My bed was right next to a window, but the night air didn't bring me any relief. No screens were supplied, so bugs and mosquitoes would come in if it was left open. We kept it ajar to take advantage of any small breeze. Both of us would have suffocated with the window fully closed. I took my chances with the mosquito attacks. We found that the best way to keep the mosquitoes out was by not keeping our lights on too long at night, because it would only attract them.

Arlene and I never seemed to be able to catch a five minute catnap because of the humid heat. I gathered up a new outfit of dry clothes and headed for a stimulating, ice-cold shower. It was then that I discovered the water was shut off at noon and not turned on again till morning.

I held on all day, imagining refreshing, icy water running down my body. Our clothes stuck to us. It wasn't hard to come to terms with the fact that changing clothes would only have the fresh ones wet again in no time. I had never had clothes drenched from sweat before, and I had a hard time adjusting to it.

It seemed worse being inside the room than outside. Arlene and I decided to just go downstairs a little early for supper. Before the meal was placed on the table, Arlene went to the corner where Father Whalen was sitting. She wanted to explain the design in her rosary pouch. He was taken aback as she positioned the little pouch in his hands.

"I understand that if you see something that seems like a miracle, you should get others to confirm it," she said.

He brought it up closer to his eyes and studied the strange detail inside. Father Whalen then turned it inside-out to get a better look. Before saying anything to her, he kissed the pouch.

"It's Our Lady holding the Baby Jesus!" he remarked.

He was astonished by the small miracle. Everyone around him got curious and came over to see what he was staring at with Arlene. It didn't take long for everyone to witness it.

It was close to 8:00 pm when we finished eating. Arlene wanted to attend the Eucharist Adoration with Father Slavko at the outside gazebo behind St. James Church.

She said, "Wait till you see the love he has for Jesus as he holds the Eucharist during Adoration."

Arriving with only ten minutes to spare, the benches were already three-quarters full. We entered from the side and were lucky to get a seat up front. We were on the side of the altar and I could only see him when he was standing. When he knelt during Adoration, he disappeared from my view.

Adoration with the Eucharist showed him in deep prayer and his eyes never left the Sacrament. He didn't appear to be aware of the hundreds of people watching and sharing this with him. He had the same expression of ecstasy on his face that the visionaries had described when they have their apparitions with Our Lady. No one and nothing else mattered around them.

Father Slavko came to the edge of the stage and held the Eucharist up in the air, making the sign of the cross with it and gradually turned it to face everyone for a special blessing. Arlene was right about the love he showed for Jesus during the worship hour.

Chapter 46
The Gifts of Medjugorje

It was now close to eleven that night as we walked back to our house from Adoration. My last stair climbing for the day was here. By now, I was so fatigued. I couldn't remember doing so much in one day. We settled in a while before changing into our pajamas. There was a small amount of water left so we could freshen up. My bed was a welcome sight.

Conversation with Arlene every night calmed me completely. It showed me where my life needed changes. Now I just have to apply it.

My life had become routine. I get up to go to work driving forty-five minutes each way; at work, I deal with tension and stress from phone sales; I arrive home around 6:00 pm, eat, shower, and then sit in front of the television until 8:00 pm. Al and I would go upstairs only to turn another television set on until the 11:00 pm news ended. I never made time to mentally unwind.

Weekends are filled with housework and errands that couldn't be done during the week. Then there are all the commitments to events, family gatherings or promised favors. Too much to do, too little time, too many missed opportunities to stop and enjoy life itself. Instead of making it fun, it became work. In a flash, Monday faces me, and it starts all over again, while I watch the clock as it dictates my schedule.

I did manage to find a place for prayer, in our guest bedroom. A statue of Our Lady had been put on a small corner table, with my rosaries and a crucifix on the wall above it. At the end of the day, I would be so tired that my only desire was to relax. Mental exhaustion would cause my prayers to be rushed or, too often, skipped completely.

Guilt would then overcome me about having pushed God aside. He's the one who brings the peace I'm searching for at the end of the day. Spending time with Him quietly, without talking, is still being in His presence. He hears us through our thoughts. I have always made simple things hard. The most important things are pushed aside, for things that can wait.

Our Lady had told the visionaries that too much time is spent in front of television. Conversations between family members have disappeared. Remotes allow us to jump from one channel to another. We watch two to three programs all at once "during the commercials." Families used to talk during these breaks.

Most of the shows are boring, distasteful, or plain silly but we watch them anyway, just to have, what we *think,* is entertainment. Television is a big part of our lives that we turn it on just to hear it while we work around the house. Instead of doing things with our children, we use it to baby sit them. Television has stopped families from doing productive things in their lives.

It has become such a habit that we don't even notice it. I can see how relationships and families can fall apart from not communicating and sharing their daily activities together. Couples that are close can drift apart without even seeing the signs. Not taking the time for one another makes us lose interest in developing the knowledge of what our kids or mates need, like or want.

Medjugorje has very little in entertainment but not once did I feel bored or lost without it. I never thought about it. My time was spent talking to strangers, taking walks to enjoy the peace it brings, in complete serenity, receiving Jesus daily through the Eucharist, going to confession to free the heaviness in my soul, attending Mass, saying a rosary or simply watching people from all over the world bonding together.

When I've spent time with Jesus and Our Lady in my thoughts, actions and prayers all day, I offer my worries up to Him. If I fall asleep saying my rosary, Our Lady will understand. My guardian angel will finish it for me.

I started to see and feel what Medjugorje is all about: inner peace with Jesus and Mary. A vacation never would have taught me this. Now I see why millions flock back to Medjugorje over and over again.

Chapter 47
Apparitions with Ivan and Mirjana

The next morning, we attended the 7:00 am Croatian Mass so I could hear the prayers and songs in their language. As we waited outside the church, Arlene and I noticed people staring up at the sky right above the church. A glorious miracle was happening before our eyes. Something was different about the sun. It was so blinding and powerful that I had to put my sunglasses on to look at it. A rainbow was forming, which seemed very strange, because no downpour had occurred. Slowly, before our eyes, it *encircled* the entire sun.

As soon as each end linked together, the sun immediately started to pulsate combining a multitude of colors consisting of pinks, blues, yellow, and purple on all sides of the sun. It gave the image of the colors exploding from it.

Arlene looked away from it for a second and remarked, "God's trying to tell us the Church is the center and core of it all."

It was a miracle bestowed on anyone who witnessed it. How could anyone doubt God after seeing this? No rainbow has ever formed a complete circle. Little signs from Heaven were being passed on to pilgrims and I wondered how many were blind to them. I went to Mass and gave thanks for being there at the right moment to receive this blessing.

Later that night, the public was invited to join Ivan on Apparition

Hill to share an apparition with our Lady at 9:40 pm. He had already had his 6:40 pm apparition, but there are times, when she appears to them again. Flashlights were required as it would be totally dark leaving. We dressed in warmer clothes and brought heavy sweatshirts in case there was be a chill in the air by the time it was over.

The climb up the hill this time was not as tough for me because the sweltering sun had begun to fade. As I stepped over the rocks in my climb, I noticed they were covered with gold specks. I wanted to take a few home since they were not ordinary rocks. I was being fussy, picking each one up and checking them over because they were all different.

On the way up, Arlene brought me to a location where, last year, there was a stone in the shape of Our Lady's face. Returning to the site, we discovered it was gone. I had witnessed the rock in a picture Arlene carried with her. My eyes searched for a stone that might be special in a form of something spiritual. I couldn't find one, so placed two stones in my backpack and continued on.

It was another beautiful, clear night. It was dusk and the sky started to display the sparkling stars in the distance. No once did we have a day with rain to hinder our activities. It was only the brutal heat that was unpleasant.

People were coming from all directions up the mountain to find a place to sit. We had a difficult time trying to find a place to sit ourselves, because of the jagged rocks. I took a pad of paper from my backpack to write in my journal. This was something I did throughout each day so I would not forget my experiences.

Not far from where we were sitting, a group of teenage boys were playing their guitars and singing. Their voices blended together and echoed off the mountain. I noticed a young girl next to me who was using her tape recorder to capture the musical sounds. Our Lady had asked Ivan to form a prayer group with the youth in Medjugorje. These were a few boys who followed him to the site to share in the apparition.

By the time we found a place to sit, it was impossible to get close to them. It was still light enough to look down the mountain at the quiet little village beneath us. The sun was going down behind the horizon and I thought, wh*en have I ever sat outside to watch the sun set?*

At 9:15 pm, an hour later, Ivan arrived with his wife, Laureen, and their daughter, who looked to be about six years old. It was hard to make them out, since the sun was gone and the darkness covered the area. As soon as Ivan and his family sat with his youth group, the group stopped singing.

Before Our Lady would descend from Heaven to appear to the visionaries, they would all start the rosary with the pilgrims joining in with the prayer.

At exactly 9:40 pm, a boy who was with Ivan announced that Our Lady was appearing. There was not a sound or movement on the hill. The world felt completely still and not one person spoke.

I was trying to comprehend the reality that Our Blessed Mother was somewhere in my presence. *She was descended from Heaven to be on Earth with us*! I closed my eyes and prayed from deep within my heart for her to bless my friends and family back home as I held the all petitions in my hand.

I selfishly wished for the chance to see or feel her. Then without being prepared to experience anything, a tremendous overpowering fragrance of roses was all around me. It was like someone put a field of roses under my nose. The aroma was so strong. Never did I find a rose on earth with such an intense scent.

Not realizing Arlene had had the same sensation, she quickly grabbed my arm. "Smell the roses? This happens when she appears!"

I knew this was gift from Our Lady. I could feel her presence in my soul from this miracle. There were no roses in the area, except near the bottom of the hill.

The apparition lasted about six minutes. The interpreter explained to the crowd what message Our Lady had told Ivan.

Ivan's exact words to the interpreter were, "Our Blessed Mother came down, smiling, happy, and with her arms extended. She prayed over us all and said she would intercede for our intentions. She prayed for the sick, and for our families back home, and asked us to pray especially for the youth. She blessed us and went up to Heaven with a radiant cross behind her."

The groups started to break up and go back down the mountain once the message was heard. I couldn't move after experiencing such a sacred occurrence. I was actually in her presence *the very moment* she appeared! How I'd longed for this experience in my life after reading about these apparitions in my Medjugorje book. It fulfilled my desire beyond anything imaginable.

Arlene sat with me, while I wrote Ivan's words down on paper. Once I completed my notes, we got up and followed the remaining group down the hill. The pilgrims had their flashlights on and the beams reminded me of fireflies as we traveled down the steep, rocky trail. There was only silence along the pathway because everyone was still feeling the holiness of the event. The scent of the roses stayed with me and I kept breathing in the fragrance so it wouldn't be lost.

Wednesday morning Arlene and I woke up at 7:00 am to have an early breakfast. We were going to see Mirjana at the Blue Cross receiving her monthly message with Our Lady. The second of each month she appears to Mirjana at this location. It was on the same roadway as Apparition Hill and only a block away. The lane leading to it was between two houses.

I desperately wanted to get as close to her as we could, but a huge crowd already formed entirely around the area where she was going to kneel. Arlene and I had to settle for sitting on the hill above Mirjana in between very thick, wild rosebushes covered with thorns. I noticed that the fragrance from the flowers attracted the bugs and bees surrounding our area.

We were there only seconds before Mirjana arrived with her interpreter. He gently motioned for the crowd to make room for her to go up to the cross. The visionaries are blessed with so much patience, enduring the hundreds of people that try to touch them.

I had to hold the brush back with my hands to get any glimpse of her. We were sitting on the ground slightly to her right. She arrived with a small, white, lace veil over her head. She went directly up to the Blue Cross without even looking at a single person in the crowd.

She expressed so much devotion trying to get there as fast as she could. Her eyes were fixed only on the cross and I did not miss the expression of love and endearment on her face as she knelt.

Like all of the visionaries, she started the rosary and the surrounding pilgrims joined her. No announcement was made that she was having her apparition but it could be seen. She suddenly was moving her lips but her words couldn't be heard.

Nothing would have distracted her. Her eyes never stopped looking above the cross while receiving her apparition. I took the petitions out of my backpack and placed them on my lap.

I gazed back at her. Tears were running down her face at the end of the apparition. The love she was feeling for Our Lady had to be beyond anything we feel for another person on Earth. It must be difficult and painful for any of them to return to our world after seeing her.

She told her interpreter what the message was for the world and left. She said Our Lady blessed all our petitions and families back home. This was my second time in Our Lady's presence. What a blessing.

Chapter 48
Climbing Cross Mountain

After Mirjana's apparition, Arlene and I headed back to the house to eat breakfast and attend the morning Mass. I felt quite tired after so many straight days of activities and late hours. Today our group was going to climb Cross Mountain. This was the biggest event I wanted to complete on my trip. It was so important for me to be able to climb to the top and look down at the little village of Medjugorje. The mountain was the most significant site in my video and I longed to climb it. My trip to Medjugorje would not be fulfilled without this accomplishment.

We ate a light meal and I became aware of my worst fear… Fibrillation. *Oh, God! Not now. Don't let this happen to me. I have to climb the mountain.* All week I'd been in perfect health. Why now? Why would Jesus let this happen?

I took a firm hold of Arlene's arm and looked at her with complete fright on my face. I pulled her aside. "I'm starting to fibrillate."

She calmly replied, "Don't panic. We'll go to Mass and pray for it to stop."

Charlie told the group that they usually climb the mountain early in the morning, but the day was going to be extremely hot, reaching close to one hundred degrees. He rescheduled to meet at 4:00 pm at the house for the climb. *This'll give me all day for the fibrillation to stop,* I prayed.

I took one of the tranquilizers the doctor had advised me to take. Usually within a half hour the problem would be gone. We both headed straight for the services. My mind wouldn't focus on anything but my heart racing. Arlene had no doubt this was how the devil worked on people to keep them away from the greatest desire that they wanted to achieve in Medjugorje.

I prayed at Mass and it didn't go away. We went back to the house and met the group on the front patio. They were in the middle of deciding who would read at each station and carry the cross going up the mountain. I volunteered to read at the second and seventh station and wondered if it would be possible to even make the trip. The more I worried about my condition, the worse my fibrillation was getting.

I said to Arlene, "I'm not going to be able to go. If I can't climb stairs at home during my attacks, how am I going to achieve climbing an actual *mountain*?"

The heat was going to make my heart problems worse, and it would take two hours in the sun to reach the summit.

Arlene was trying to get me to relax. By now everyone in the group knew of my dilemma. I went upstairs to my bedroom to get some rest, hoping it would go away. Arlene went shopping so I could be alone to rest.

I slept for an hour and after opening my eyes, I could still feel the fibrillation. My clothes were soaked from sleeping in the heat. No more water was available to take a shower and it frustrated me. If I could have cooled off, it would have taken some of the stress off my heart. This was the worst day of the week reaching the highest temperatures of ninety.

Supper was going to be at 3:00 pm that day because of the scheduled journey. I wouldn't be able to eat a full meal before our climb. The food would not digest in time and it could cause difficulty in breathing from exerting myself so soon. *Oh Lord, what a test.*

Burying my embarrassment, I went up to Father Whalen and told him of my condition. I expressed my fear of not being able to go with the group. He felt the same as Arlene, agreeing it was the devil working to keep me from fulfilling the climb.

Father asked if the group could pray over me. I told him it would be welcomed. Everyone held hands and circled around me. As Father prayed, I realized the prayer was Anointing of the Sick, said at the last rites. I heard the words, "To heal and forgive sins since your last confession." One has to prepare themselves for death like Jakov said. Father Whalen continued to bless everyone in the group for their trip to Cross Mountain.

One gentleman came over to me and said he could relate to what I was going through. During his first trip to Medjugorje, he'd had an angina attack trying to climb the mountain and swore he was going to die. Half way to the top, it somehow passed.

Arlene suggested taking a taxi to the mountain to avoid anymore walking than was necessary. Cross Mountain was not that far from the house, but walking in between my heart skipping and racing was not only exhausting, but it was hard to breathe. I got into the taxi thinking about what a huge mistake it was to do any physical activity in my condition. I felt that pushing myself would only cause a serious need to go to the hospital.

We drove past the rest of the group walking and within two minutes we arrived at the foot of the hill. My fears rose higher. The climb up the mountain was not gradual. It was steeper than Apparition Hill. At the foot of the hill, there were thick sticks that resembled staffs to help people with the climb. I took one incase it was needed.

I had concentrated so much on my heart troubles that I had forgot about bringing water with me. I looked around and noticed everyone else had bottles connected to their belts. This was so important with the two hours of climbing that would be facing me. I tried desperately to hide my hands: they were shaking from nerves. My heart bounced inside my chest, out of normal rhythm. It was difficult even to talk. I fought back tears from fright and stress. If I broke down and cried, I would lose complete control of the situation.

Another man in our group came up to me and said, "Try going to just one or two stations and then come back down."

I knew he meant well, but how could I go that far, and then turn around? I *had* to climb to the top.

Arlene took me aside, "Watch me. I'm going to show you how to go up the mountain. Take each step very slowly, like you're actually in slow motion. Do not rush it." She learned this technique with her climb last year. "People make the mistake of trying to go up too fast."

Arlene stayed in front of me so I could not pass her. Slowly, I put one foot in front of the other. We would take a step and then hesitate to almost a complete stop before taking the next one. I could feel my heart beating in my throat. I was wondering why on Earth I was doing this with my heart problem. *Was I insane?*

I had studied the picture of Cross Mountain in my book over and over again. I imagined myself sitting on top, absorbing the whole wonder of this miracle in Medjugorje.

We arrived at the second station and it was my turn to read. I said each word slowly and steadily so no one would see how out of breath I was. The group began to depart for the next station when a man came up to me and poured his bottled-water all over my head. He actually gave up his whole supply of water to give me relief from the heat.

This man didn't think twice about what he had lost for himself. His only concern was to make me comfortable. Being so touched by his kindness, I took his hands and gave a smile with my eyes full of tears. No words had to be exchanged between us.

I kept pulling air into my chest, trying to control the fibrillation. I needed to rest but did not want to fall behind. Finally, a point came where I decided to pull away mentally from just thinking about myself. I started to offer my suffering up for the Souls in Purgatory. It seemed more important to sacrifice my discomfort than to concentrate on it.

I knew Father Whalen had just given me the last rites to start my journey and my confession had been heard a few days before, so my soul had been cleansed from sin. If God decided to take me during my climb, I felt spiritually ready.

As ridiculous as it may sound, I wondered more about how my family would get my body back home. It was crazy how many things went through my mind in minutes while I tried to reach the top of the mountain. I started to comprehend that it is not about our bodies: Jesus is only interested in our souls. That's where all our love and faith is contained.

My father entered my thoughts. He had wanted to travel to Medjugorje as much as I did. Eight years had passed since his death. Leona had prayed the rosary and attended Mass for him every single morning for over a year. She received peace in knowing he was home with God.

I wanted the same peace within my soul. *Why else would I be here? What was the reason for my calling? This had to be at least one of them. God, if he's not with you now, please take him when I get to the top of the mountain. Let this be my journey for him spiritually.* This was going to be my gift to Dad. I started to ignore my discomfort and kept my eyes looking up at the cross on top of the mountain which was facing me. I felt the presence of Jesus in my heart.

I read again at the seventh station and started up the hill. It wasn't until we reached the eleventh station that I felt my heart jump back into a normal rhythm. My pain was replaced by a peaceful feeling. Once I had put my life into God's hands, my health was restored. *Why did I doubt Him?*

Tears overcame me once I realized what Jesus was trying to teach me. I truly believe that at one time or another, we will all suffer, whether it is mentally or physically. It's our punishment from our sins: like Adam and Eve. Jesus waits for us to offer up our suffering and trust in Him. With my heart problem gone, it was like a fire was under me to get to the peak.

Feeling totally worn out, I said to Arlene, "I'm fine now. It left as soon as I offered my suffering up."

She hugged me, looking relieved.

Nearing my final steps, the huge cross appeared in front of me. Reaching the top, I saw our group talking. They had been proud making the two hour journey.

I passed by them and left Arlene to be by myself. I walked by the famous, enormous cross and went straight to a small, stained wooden cross completely on the other side. It was weather-beaten and stood about two feet tall. I felt a strong force leading me there to kneel and pray.

I wondered why there, instead of falling at the large concrete cross, the one I had longed to reach. I felt very humble and small looking at this cross that was completely isolated. Jesus had led a simple life and I felt a very private connection to Him at this location.

After my prayers, I knew in my heart that my father was in Heaven. I received the peace that Leona already had. Maybe that was why she wasn't called and I was. *Did I need this journey to Medjugorje to find this peace?*

When I ended giving thanks to Jesus for helping me finish my journey, I looked for Arlene. Such a remarkable woman; she knew when to let me be by myself. A week's friendship and we both understood the importance of being alone to become connected to the Holy Spirit. That's the secret: being alone in prayer. If you are patient, you *will* feel Him.

Arlene and I sat together silently on the Cross Mountain steps looking down at the village. My eyes and heart were awestruck witnessing the sight I had longed to see. Nothing else on Earth could have been more of a blessing or gift from Jesus and Mary.

Our group gathered in front of the giant cross to take pictures. There was so much peace in my body and mind that I had no desire to leave my spot to join them. The pictures were in my heart. I knew what was witnessed would never be replaced or topped by any other trip, not even Hawaii.

An hour passed before Arlene and I joined friends to start down Cross Mountain. I picked up my staff and waved my left hand in the onward motion like Moses for them to follow me. It was hard to believe that I was now skipping down the path.

Everyone laughed after sharing in my struggle coming up the mountain. They saw me joyful after a long journey of pain and suffering. Maybe it is similar to the same agony we have to go through before entering into Heaven. My misery showed me God's love. The most important experience of my trip was accomplished. Satan was once again defeated!

Once we reached the bottom of the mountain, we all walked to a restaurant directly across the street. Everyone refreshed themselves with cold drinks. Exhaustion took over after fighting to control my physical and mental state of health throughout the whole day. Other pilgrims started to walk back to the houses or called for taxis. I joined in sharing a ride because my knees felt like rubber. There was no more energy left in me to walk the short distance back.

Chapter 49
Final Day in Medjugorje

I woke up Friday morning, facing my last full day at Medjugorje. My flight was leaving Saturday and already the sadness and depression could be felt deep within me. I went to the 10:00 am Mass absolutely heartbroken knowing there wouldn't be another morning to sit in this sacred church. How could I go back to my church, with only one priest on the altar and many empty pews?

Arlene and I finally decided to visit the gift stores to look for holy items. The store behind the church caught my eye with the beautiful statues displayed in front of it. I made sure everyone in the family was going to receive a rosary.

As we walked around the village, Eddie came upon us with a warm and proud smile on his face.

"I brought something really special for the two of you," he replied.

He had come across a medal that was the exact image of Mary holding baby Jesus that was embedded into Arlene's rosary pouch. The medal would always remind us of the gift given to Arlene from Our Lady.

After shopping, I decided to go back to the house early and start packing. This way there would be no anxiety of having to think about it all day. I climbed the stairs with no enthusiasm. The combination of not wanting to leave Medjugorje and knowing Arlene and Eddie were staying longer made it hard to accept. After getting my things in order, we spent the day praying and watching the pilgrims going in and out of St. James Church.

Supper felt very special, since it was my last night. The dining area was extremely noisy with everyone talking all at once about their week's events. Individuals were passing out their names, addresses and phone numbers on paper. I could now understand how friendships developed on a pilgrimage.

After a very relaxing meal, Penny, from Denver, joined us for a walk around the area. She and Arlene had met on last year's trip to Medjugorje. The hot sun was setting and there was a motionless feeling in the air. My eyes were acting like a camera, trying to take pictures of every inch of Medjugorje so it would last forever in my mind.

Arlene wanted to show me the cemetery at the far end of St. James Church. The graves were all above the ground, encased in cement monuments like the ones we had passed as we had come into the village. It was peaceful and serene, with only the sound of the birds. The three of us started making our way back when suddenly the aroma of roses filled the air.

I stopped dead in my tracks, "Oh! Smell the roses?"

There were no roses in the area. Penny and Arlene didn't smell any. It was the same strong scent as on Apparition Hill when Our Lady was appearing to Ivan.

Arlene just smiled, "It must be a gift just for you from the Blessed Mother before you leave."

It was so difficult to keep my emotions together with the sorrow that was starting to fill my whole body. I wanted to wrap-up the whole village and take it home. I knew the same old habits and problems not found in Medjugorje would be facing me on my return.

I knew deep down that there would be a struggle with television consuming my life again. There are many decent programs to watch but most sitcoms or movies contained nudity or suggestive scenes. Swearing is sneaking its way into television. When we were young, our mouths were washed out with soap using these words. Bathroom scenes have become important to add to movies while people have conversations.

Young children are giving up their virginity to be popular. A virgin is laughed at today. Men and women want to know what the goods are before they marry. In the olden days, we used to hear no one wanted "damaged goods." People have sex whenever they want and with whomever thinking there is nothing wrong with it. Desires are filled without even thinking twice about it. Walking down the aisle in *white* was special and had meaning. The wedding night was a shared moment between two people who waited with love and eagerness, and had saved their virginity for their special partners.

Drugs and alcohol are another crutch people use to try and solve their problems. Getting a high supposedly puts the world on a back burner. People wake up not knowing how to deal with problems, or they want to lose themselves in drugs to avoid solving them. They have no knowledge that healing can come through prayer and turning to God.

Pregnancies are bringing so many innocent and unwanted babies into the world and abortions are just another way out of responsibilities. Divorces are such a normal thing today that people don't think a thing about them. Children are brought up with only one parent and we don't think this is important. Marriage is entered into with the feeling if it doesn't work, get divorced; no big deal. Innocent people are being raped and killed. Infants are being beaten, abused mentally or physically and brought up with no love or security.

There are many good and decent children and adults caught up in these problems. Wrong choices have been made or someone has forced themselves on the innocent victims.

There has always been violence in our world and issues with our children struggling to make the right decisions, but as time has gone on, it gets worse. We need to bring our religious beliefs back into our lives and practice them as a family.

No wonder God is making demands. It's only a matter of time when He will make a decision and take action on our sins. God will not have to ask our permission or acceptance like we look for in our children. He is giving us choices, and either we do not see them, or we choose to ignore the warnings. When the time comes, it will not matter if you do not believe in the existence of God. *He Is* and the events will happen whether people believe or not. Pray so God will help you feel Him.

I ached to go home and have our world turn back the way it was in the early years. Let us enter marriages without the sex first, go down the church aisle in white for a reason, say no to a child if it is not in their best interest or safety, stop trying to be friends to our children and just be parents, send children out of the room during adult conversations, teach our families to respect someone who may not be the same race or faith, spend more time with family, and let us close the businesses and malls to give Sundays back to Jesus. We have to save our children. They grow up with what they see and hear from the adults. It starts with us.

"However, take care and be earnestly on your guard not to forget the things which your own eyes have seen, nor let them slip from your memory as long as you live, but teach them to your children and to your children's children" (Deuteronomy 4:9).

I believe that Our Lady wants all the pilgrims, who had come to Medjugorje, to go home and spread peace and help to convert others so they will return to their faith. Medjugorje shows us in our hearts what is really important in our lives and not to focus on the material things. When people back home see us doing good for others, they may want to follow. We have to keep God's name in our speech, actions and writings.

Visionaries all over the world are trying to save us by informing the world what they are actually seeing and hearing from Our Lady or Jesus Himself. They have seen everything that is here and beyond. If we listen and do what is asked of us, which is not much, we will end up at the same doors where the visionaries will be at the end of time. What more could we ask for than to spend our lives with God in peace and happiness after our death?

We all enter this world alone and we will leave it alone. It's up to each individual to decide what to do with his or her own life because no one else can decide this for us. No one can save you from Hell except yourself. If you believe in God, your soul will be saved. The existence of God and Heaven will not disappear just because you may not believe in them. God's own words are, *"I Am...That I Am" (Exodus, 3.14).*

Medjugorje has given me a renewal of life. Time will tell me why I was called here. I will have to sit and listen quietly for God to talk to me when I'm alone.

Nothing visible or earthshaking hit me this week, at least not on the outside. I felt it deep within my soul. My pilgrimage showed me how I can live without the material things. This, I think this is the answer. We belong to God and talk to Him in our souls. Believing and putting our trust into His hands, will bring us closer to Him.

We have to open our hearts every single day, with no fear, for Him to enter our souls and lead us to Heaven. You don't believe? That's all right...Tell Him. God already knows it and everything else about us. He is aware of our wants, needs and desires. Prayer is just talking to God as one would a friend or a parent. Ask the Holy Spirit to come and help you understand it all. Pray, Pray, Pray and you will feel Him. *"God is our refuge and our strength an ever-present help in distress" (Psalm 46:2).*

Prayer slows down your fast-paced life. Difficulties in decision-making will fall in place with the answers. Peace will come to you and turmoil and despair will leave you. We have to come to the realization soon that our time on Earth is short, but our life after death is forever. Where do you want to spend it? There are two choices at the time of our death: Heaven or Hell. Until our world ends, God is merciful by giving us Purgatory.

I walked quietly back to the village, realizing how much I had learned in a week. I had not noticed until now. We headed for the restaurant for our last ice cream sundae treat. The café was full to capacity because so many were leaving the next morning. No one wanted the night to end. The three of us could not find a seat until Eddie motioned that he had saved a spot.

The restaurant had no enclosure and it was enjoyable to sit outside late at night under the stars. The deafening laughter and voices were strident from all the pent-up excitement and the feelings of restlessness that was here in all of us.

I didn't want the night to end, but fatigue was catching up with me. Every day was long. We woke around 7:00 am and rarely went to bed earlier than midnight. Once I hit the bed, my trip was over.

Finally around eleven, I headed upstairs to my room. It was a relief to know my clothes were already packed. The bus was going to arrive around seven, so breakfast would be early. The nightly conversation between the two of us was not long because of my need for sleep. We tried to squeeze as much talk as we could before drifting off.

Chapter 50
Leaving Medjugorje

I woke up at 5:00 am to the sound of suitcases bouncing down the stairs. The noise acted as an alarm clock for those of us about to leave Medjugorje. The men in the group were busy collecting the suitcases that had been left outside each door so they could be put into the bottom bus compartments.

I tried to look happy, but the sorrow was absolutely engulfing me. *How am I going to leave?* I asked God to forgive me for being so self-centered in wanting to stay longer.

Arlene joined me for an early breakfast that was prepared for the ones leaving. I had no real appetite, but ate a boiled egg with a piece of Italian bread. I put an apple in my backpack since it was going to be a long trip home. There was complete commotion with everyone running around the dining area, saying goodbye to the others staying behind and to the family who had served us the whole week.

Every step towards to the bus was forced, and my smile felt like it was pasted on. After all the pieces of luggage were counted, the group started up the bus steps to depart. Arlene and I kissed each other goodbye, acting like the torment was not bothering either of us. The tears were ready to come, so I hugged her fast and went on the bus.

I sat by a window and looked out at the village for one last time. I was leaving a place with so much love and tranquility. I waved to Arlene until the bus disappeared around the corner.

We passed St. James Church and I thought, *If only I could cry to let this pain escape—it was choking me.* I had now learned what the true feelings were after a pilgrimage and had come to know why everyone wanted to return. I was leaving and already wondered if I would ever come back.

As we started to pull out of the village, I could see Cross Mountain in the distance to my left. I gazed out the window and lovingly spoke to Our Lady, "You called and gave me this wonderful gift, and now it is hard to leave. Please help me bring this knowledge home to my friends and family."

I stared at the holy mountain, knowing my biggest dream had come true. I was now comfortable with leaving because I felt my father deep within me. Dad's presence would always be in Medjugorje. "You're home now, Dad. I did this for both of us. Serenity will always follow me knowing that you're in Heaven with our Father."

I had come to Medjugorje thinking I needed answers after my father's death, but now I realized it was just a healing heart that was needed in order to be able to say goodbye. *"Have no anxiety at all, but in everything, by prayer and petition, with thanksgiving, make your request known to God. Then the peace of God that surpasses all understanding will guard your hearts and minds in Christ Jesus."* (Philippians 4:6-7)

We were an hour and a half into the ride to the airport when the bus came to a complete stop. It was still not completely daybreak, and I couldn't see what location we were at. The bus driver opened the door for a soldier to come aboard. Since I had sat at the back of the bus, I couldn't hear what the driver and soldier were saying to each other up front.

As the soldier started down the middle of the aisle, I notice he had a rifle over his shoulder. When he came closer to my seat, I realized he was not an American by his uniform. This had to be official business, because we were all asked to hand our passports over to him.

I looked out the window and noticed three more soldiers with rifles outside the bus. I felt uneasy. After he had collected all the passports, he went out to the other soldiers. I quickly leaned over to a man across the aisle and asked if this was a normal procedure.

The gentleman explained, "I've been here a few times and never had it happen."

I later learned we were at the International boarder crossing between Bosnia-Herzegovina and Croatia. This is where passports are required to be shown as requested. I thought that maybe they stopped buses at random.

Within minutes, the bus started to move again, and the passports were passed back to us. I felt foolish being scared over normal procedures.

The sun was just coming up and the scenery was, again, beautiful along the Adriatic seacoast. The bus went at a slow pace, bouncing over the same unpaved roads we had traveled coming into Medjugorje.

I became conscious of the fact that I loved my family, but the love I felt for Medjugorje, was not something from this earth—it was from Heaven. It's a love that became so deep inside my heart and soul, I wanted to reach out and embrace it above anything else in my life-even my loved ones. I felt the closeness of Jesus and Our Lady more than I ever could have imagined.

Medjugorje is a *sampler* of Heaven. We learn and feel what awaits us if we turn to peace, love, and worship. We should treat all strangers as though they were Jesus standing in front of us. If I had a choice as to where I would like to be at the time of my death, it would be here in this little village—it's the closest I will ever be to Paradise.

Once we left Split, there would only be one layover at the Newark Airport. I spent the eight hours on the flight reading books about Medjugorje. I felt totally lost, traveling back without Arlene. She had become my dearest friend. A few hours of sleep would have been a blessing, but my insides were on high speed, reminiscing about my week's experiences.

I sat back and re-thought about all I'd learned on the pilgrimage. The main messages the visionaries passed onto us were conversion and not to wait for the last secret to unfold. *So why aren't we listening to the warning signs?*

There are hundreds of unbelievers who have not yet come to know God. The Blessed Mother is telling us to turn back to prayer, penance, and Mass. These warnings have been delivered by her years before and since her apparitions in Medjugorje. These messages are meant for all the people God has created, from every religion. I believe we were called to Medjugorje to become disciples of God when we depart. It's our calling to spread the word about the chastisements and save souls before it's too late.

The Holy Spirit was deep in my soul, and I wanted to touch every person who was going to come in contact with me, so they would believe as much as I did.

I was thankful that our flight to New Jersey felt fast. As we approached to land onto the runway, the plane came in with the left wing slanted towards the ground.

Everyone was saying out loud, "Straighten out…Straighten out."

Smiles from relief were exchanged along with nervous laughs and loud claps as we touched down safely. Suddenly, passengers started to crowd the aisle and grab their belongings from the overhead bins. They were already standing, before the plane had come to a complete stop at the terminal. I wondered why they had stood so soon, with nowhere to go. We were now jammed together without being able to move.

People from our group were going in different directions leaving Newark to go home. Many were saying goodbye extremely fast so the others could catch their flight to Boston and other connections.

As I boarded my last flight, I took comfort in knowing there was only an hour and a half left before Al would meet me at Logan Airport in Boston. I couldn't wait for the reunion. He would probably not be able to see the changes in me: they were all in my soul. How would he understand? He is not spiritual and would never be able to comprehend the blessings that were given to me. I was not the same person returning home. So much of me was left in Medjugorje.

When I came off the plane, I could see Al waiting at the gate. We had been separated for a week and my heart melted when I saw his smile.

My embrace came from the heart as we hugged and kissed. I had become an independent flyer.

Instantly, things around me started to revert to what I considered to be normal but fast-paced. People started pushing, shoving and bumping into us as they rushed to meet their scheduled flights, or as they tried to get into line to collect their baggage. No one cared that they were cutting in front of others. As they tried to retrieve their suitcases, swears were heard from the impatient travelers who had to wait, or search for their lost belongings.

I had just left Medjugorje, where there was nothing but constant peace and respect for strangers sharing their space. Someone in need was helped without even thinking twice about it. There was no rushing or schedule needed in Medjugorje. The village had only the sounds of prayer, music from St. James Church, and the echo of birds. My eyes filled, thinking about what I had just left behind.

Al put my large suitcase into the trunk of the car and we drove out of the airport. The traffic was bumper to bumper through the Callahan Tunnel. Al joined the maniac drivers on Route 93 to go home to Rochester. Cars were passing on the right and left of us. One minute he had to drive at a high rate of speed to keep up with the traffic and then we were in a line of cars showing nothing but brake lights as far as the eye could see.

How can so many people be on the road at once? Where are they all going? What's their rush? *I don't want to be back here.* Al would never identify with what I was feeling. All the muscles in my neck were tight as I watched the traffic coming at us from all directions. I felt sick to my stomach watching how drivers became insane behind the wheel of a car. People would cut us off, give the finger, show hatred in their eyes, and swear at us.

I could feel the wonderful peace and tranquility that I had brought back come to an end. At the same time this was all happening, Al was smiling and talking to me but I was not even listening to what was being said. He had no awareness of all this turmoil. I tried to study the life I was returning to. How did the world get this way without me ever noticing it?

The further we got from Boston, the further I felt from Medjugorje. I wanted to go back where this commotion did not exist. This was not the time to explain this to Al, so I sat back and tried to go along with the fast flow.

Chapter 51
Changes in and Around My Life

Sunday morning, I got up to see a new addition in our backyard next to the fireplace. Just as Arlene predicted, Al had bought a beautiful statue of Our Lady ensconced in a grotto. He was very proud of himself. My happiness only added to his delight. He described all the running around that occurred at different locations until he found one with the perfect beautiful details on her face. I was touched that he had searched so hard for the right statue to present to me.

Returning back to work filled me with a sense of loss. I struggled to get back to the working environment. I felt caged for eight hours when, before I'd been free to pray wherever and whenever without any outside distractions. I came to understand how people gave up all their worldly goods to live in Medjugorje. My peace and calmness were disappearing. It was now easy for me to realize why people went back repeatedly.

Gifts that I had purchased on my trip were passed out to my close friends at work. I gave out medals, prayer cards and pictures. The girls took me out to lunch because they wanted to hear about my journey. I couldn't believe everyone's excitement. We all had different religious beliefs, but I explained how Medjugorje was for people of all faiths. God wants all his children around the whole world to be saved.

After lunch, I rushed over to see Maryanne and asked how Todd was doing. I feared he might have passed away while I was gone.

"The doctors are amazed," she replied. "He's back working at the pizza store and joined a baseball league. He's also making plans to marry."

My first thought was, *another miracle like the ones Dad had talked about.*

Debbi Bettencourt was excited when she came into my office a few months after my return. She informed me she was pregnant. This had been her request to Our Lady in her petition. She had never told anyone that there had been a few miscarriages in the past. In time she delivered twin girls named Maddy and Ally—a double blessing. I called them the *Medjugorje Miracle Babies.*

Val Poitras, our daughter Lynne's father-in-law, had his prostate cancer cured after giving me his petition. His wife, Georgette, had placed the silver medal that I'd given her on the claw clasp of her sterling silver bracelet. Within days the clasp turned gold. A jeweler tried buffing the gold off. He had no explanation as to why he could not return it to the original silver.

Less than a year after my trip, the chain links of my father's traveling rosaries turned gold. I called Leona to tell her about my discovery as soon as it happened.

Before I could share the excitement, she cut me off. Her voice was shaking as she explained an event to me, "You're the only one I can tell this story to because no one else would believe me. I had the most incredible experience just now."

She had been under a lot of stress with the business and feared she was on the verge of a breakdown. Living in Buzzards Bay running the lumber business without Bob, while he lived in Punxsutawney, Pennsylvania, running their mattress store, put a lot of strain on her. They had been doing this for five years.

She continued, "I was sitting in the back room doing the bookkeeping, and my nerves were ready to jump out of my body. Without any warning, I was physically lifted into another place. It looked like Jerusalem and I was standing in a crowd on a cobble street.

It wasn't a dream, I was living it. A man passed by and brushed his gown against me. It was Jesus! I did not see His face because His back was to me. I felt Him. His gown was the same cream color as Dad's rosaries and His hair was long. As soon as the gown touched me, a tremendous peace came over me. It seemed like all the pressure was lifted from me. I actually felt Jesus! Please don't think I'm crazy," she said with uncontrollable sobs.

Once she calmed down and stopped crying, I said, "Leona, I believe you. Let me tell you about Dad's rosaries." When the story was completed, I continued, "Isn't it odd for our two supernatural events to have happened on the same day?"

When I saw her a few days later, I gave her our father's rosaries. She kept them a short time, claiming I was meant to keep them because of the changes occurring in my life since Dad's death.

September 11, 1999, our daughter Carol, agreed with the family it was time to get her son, Jordan (nine years old), and daughter, Julia (seven years old) baptized. She and Bill had been separated and she was living with us. Al's other daughter, Lynne, and her husband Ron, were the Godparents.

Monsignor Perry from the St. John Neumann Church in East Freetown was going to celebrate the religious sacrament. It was the first time we had entered this church. I attended St. Rose of Lima Church in Rochester alone, since Al was not going to Mass.

When we entered the narthex, I noticed a picture of Our Lady on the wall. It was the same as the ones sold in Medjugorje. I looked at Al and said, "This is going to be our church." I felt deep down that this was a sign.

As the baptism proceeded with Monsignor Perry, I prayed deeply, "Please, Holy Spirit, come down upon all of us. Bless our whole family and bring them back to church. Help Al receive the desire to start attending Mass with me. Let Carol get through her painful divorce." There were so many family members I was praying for to return back to God; my brothers, sons, daughters.

Al liked Monsignor Perry right away. He also loved the fact that the church had air conditioning. Lynne and Ron mentioned that they attended the 8:00 am Mass every Sunday and invited us to join them. Right away my prayers were answered when Al and Carol both showed an interest in going.

What a joyous morning, when Sunday arrived and everyone was getting ready for church. George Martin was a parishioner who passed out the weekly bulletin at the door. He became a very important person in our lives, pulling us closer to this church.

It was such a blessed gift to see the whole family sitting together in the pew. When it came time for Holy Communion, everyone started down the aisle to receive. No one was conscious that they had not been to confession. I knew it had been years since Al went. This was not the time to explain this to them so I put it in God's hands and let it go. The last thing I wanted to do was to turn them away from church when they were turning back to their faith.

Coffee and donuts were served in the church hall weekly, after Mass. Monthly breakfasts were also offered. Al was really impressed, thinking this would be something good for the family to share. He especially liked the idea of coffee since he drank so much of it. I laughed. *If it takes coffee and air conditioning to get him to church...let it be God.* All the parishioners were friendly and sincere about caring for others. I prayed my husband would continue to go to church and not have this be a one-time event, attended out of curiosity.

One summer, George invited us to help out with the yearly church chicken barbecue. To my surprise, Al accepted, without thinking twice about it. George enlisted us into the St. John Neumann's Couples Club. What a wonderful group of people. Once a month, a committee would schedule entertainment for the members. We would take numerous trips to the Foxwood Casino, shows, dinners, bowling and our summers ended routinely at Chuck and Julie Millington's yard in August for a pool party.

Father's Day, we attended Mass and were honored to be chosen to bring the offering up to the altar. I couldn't believe such a blessing was being bestowed on us this special day. As we presented the offering to the priest, I could not hide the tears of happiness. Medjugorje was working its graces and miracles on us as a couple. Never would I have pictured Al going to church, never mind going down the aisle with the offering, on Father's Day, no less.

Unexpectedly, one night, Carol decided to go back to her husband in Maine. It had been a year of constant court battles. She gave us the story that she was taking the kids out to supper and a late movie. They did not come home that night.

I told Al my vibes were strong that she went back to Bill with the kids. This would have been the second time she had left and returned to him. I'd been praying the rosary, day after day, for her to get her life together and for God to bring someone loving and decent into her life.

Al called me at work with the news that Carol was back in Maine with Bill. It affected me so much that I had to leave work. We had been trying to help her put the pieces back in her life…and it was over again.

When this happened, I questioned my own faith: why did God let this happen? Why did she go back to him? This was not what I'd been praying for in her life. It took a few months for me to realize that God did answer my prayers. He did it in His time and way.

I prayed for her to be happy and she was. It just didn't happen the way I wanted it. My way was with someone else, so she would not be hurt again. I had to let go and let God decide what was best for her. After all, wasn't that what I was praying for?

On November 24, 2000, Father Slavko Barbaric died, at the age of fifty-eight, in Medjugorje. He was saying the rosary, leading a multitude of pilgrims on the journey up Cross Mountain. Calmly, he had sat down to rest and then had passed away. For nineteen and a half years, he had traveled throughout the whole world, teaching prayer and the love of Jesus and Mary. What a loss to all of us.

In December of 2000, Arlene, Al and I went to LaSalette in Attleboro to see the Christmas decorations. We were not aware that Bishop Sean O'Malley from Fall River was going to say a Mass and give the shrine a blessing before turning on the lights for the holiday.

This was Al's first time hearing him speak. He loved the bishop's gentleness and his strong, clear voice. Bishop O'Malley reminded me of Jesus when he came down the aisle wearing his sandals and carrying a staff.

It was a Millennium Mass and we were told if confession was made before the New Year, all our sins of the past would be forgiven. Arlene and I went but Al stayed behind. I had to let him handle his own inner healing.

The next week, Al secretly went back to LaSalette Shrine to have his confession heard, his first time in over thirty years. Our Lady was working miracles beyond my imagination with my husband. *How powerful is prayer?*

Chapter 52
Todd's Death

In May of 2000, Maryanne came to my office with the sad news that Todd had died from cancer. I was so saddened after praying so hard in Medjugorje for this stranger who had entered my heart. I accepted it as God's will.

His wake was in Taunton which was about a forty-minute drive. I had to attend for reasons beyond me. I'd never been to a wake where I didn't know the deceased or a member of the family. During the whole drive, I kept debating about turning around and going back home. *No one was going to know me.*

I entered the Capro-Hathaway Funeral Home parking lot and the late afternoon sun was still strong. Groups of young adults were sitting outside talking. They looked shocked and heartbroken over losing their friend.

I opened the door to the funeral home and tried to blend into the line leading into the room where the casket was positioned. An easel at the doorway held pictures of his short-lived life with friends and family. Todd had only been in his early twenties.

I wanted to see what he looked like to connect to him too—but it was a closed ceremony. I was disappointed that I would be unable to see his face. When I knelt in front of the casket, I noticed a picture of him positioned on top of it. His red hair caught my attention.

When Todd got married, I had bought a picture from LaSalette Shrine as a wedding gift. It showed a young boy in dungarees wearing a t-shirt. His eyes were closed as he leaned the back of his limp body and head against the chest of Jesus. His hand was hanging down by his side, holding a hammer. Jesus was holding the boy up in His arms.

Instantly, I saw Todd as the boy in the picture. With his cancer, he had had the same need for God's strength to hold him up. The boy in the picture and Todd both had red hair. Maryanne said his new wife could not look at the picture because she only saw death. His mother and father took it and hung it up in their home. They had a positive reaction to it because it filled their own personal needs.

I was now before a boy who was no longer a stranger in my soul. After saying a short prayer, I went over to his wife to introduce myself. She demonstrated no interest in me as I tried explaining who I was. At that moment, she was only experiencing personal pain and was in a confused state with a stranger facing her.

When I mentioned taking the envelope with Todd's hair to Medjugorje, I heard someone in the background say, "I know her."

His mother stepped out from the family line and took my hand, introducing herself. I could feel the emotions from the bottom of her heart, as she thanked me for coming. We had never met, but Maryanne had connected us by telling me about his mother's prayers throughout his prolonged illness. I expressed how very sorry I was with his passing.

She sincerely replied, "God gave us two more years with him after your trip."

His father could not come up to me but I went and gently held his hands before going out the door. I hoped my appearance gave his parents some comfort, knowing I cared about their loss.

It was when I got into the car that closure was made with Todd. This was my way of letting go and saying goodbye to him. God has His reasons beyond our ever knowing why or when certain souls are called back to Him earlier in life than others.

Chapter 53
Church Sex Scandal

Since the mid 1990's, more than 130 people came forward regarding sexual abuse in the Catholic Church. It was kept quiet and very low-keyed by Church officials. By January 6, 2002, it was blown wide open by the media. When the television was turned on, the newspaper was read, or when we listened to the radio, it was a topic discussed by everyone.

This was when I realized why Mirjana, the visionary from Medjugorje, told us that Our Lady was asking the world to pray for our priests. That was back in 1998 and she knew how strong Satan had become and that the Church would be tested.

The public and parishioners wanted punishment to all priests involved in these legal proceedings. Victims demanded to be compensated, along with having the priests publicly admit to their actions and to ask for forgiveness.

Many were angry and repulsed by the Church. Officials had not only known about the sexual abuse, but had done nothing about it. Priests could've been sent to monasteries for solitary punishment, with heavy counseling, not only for the offender, but also for the victim. If they had made these changes, it would have helped prevent priests from having any further contact with children. Instead, they positioned them in other parishes, only to have them repeat the same offenses.

Many Catholics have refused to return to the Church or give any support since this has happened. The biggest loss for individuals walking away from the Church is their failure to practice their faith. They have deprived themselves of receiving the Body and Blood of Jesus Christ during Holy Communion. He is the One who gives us life.

We have all lost in this tragedy. Some priests have been convicted. The innocent ones will be condemned by the public for years to come. Their responsibilities have been taken away from them; many were put into early retirement, others left the priesthood on their own. Many stepped away from the church that they loved. Victims were left feeling anger towards the Church and priests. They struggle with returning to Mass and keeping their belief in God.

Beautiful churches were now left with no priests to celebrate Mass. All too many have closed. Parishioners had looked at the closings as hassles and many avoided traveling long distances to a new church. Others just miss the church they attended for years and stopped going completely. What has the scandal done—it has stopped many from having the will to worship.

We can't blame God for these sinners. Priests are human. They have the free will to choose right from wrong. Those who were tempted into sex abuse had come under the control of Satan, like any of us. He attacks the weak.

Satan has the power and control over people who have no desire to return to church. He is keeping them from receiving graces from the Holy Eucharist and the Holy Spirit, which gives us the strength to handle the everyday hardships. Most importantly, Satan is keeping them from being in a holy state before their time of death. He doesn't want anyone to go to Heaven. The more we pray, the stronger our faith becomes and the closer we get to Jesus.

We shouldn't allow such an evil spirit to take special blessings away from us. Our best protection is uniting again in the House of God. Nothing in this world will make the Church fall. When the chastisements are over, Our Lady has told the visionaries that Satan will no longer reign. She will triumph over him. If a certain church, or priest, makes someone uncomfortable, we should search one where we find peace.

We are all sinners in this life. If someone falls, pray for them. We have our own sins to ask God to forgive. There's going to be a judgment day and no one will slip by Jesus. Forgive, so He will forgive you.

Chapter 54
Eucharistic Ministry

On June 22, 2002, I became a Eucharistic Minister for the St. John Neumann Church in East Freetown. I never truly felt worthy to hold the Body and Blood of Jesus in my hands. Al was already a collector at the 8:00 am Mass. We never missed going to church, unless we were too sick. If I'm not able to attend, Al gets up and goes by himself, instead of using it as an excuse to stay home. I don't think he realizes that his involvement in church activities and services, are blessings from opening his heart to allow Jesus to come into it.

As time went on, I started to become uncomfortable at the altar. It wasn't from shyness being in front of everyone on the altar, but a strong inner soul feeling that it might not be right to serve the Body and Blood of Jesus like priests.

During confession one Saturday, I mentioned these emotions. The priest told me even they do not feel worthy. I was confused, wondering if it was God telling me this, or if the devil was trying to get me to walk away from this responsibility and lose the closeness to Jesus. I tried to ignore this uneasiness for a year.

June 28, 2003, Arlene, Al and I were invited by Eddie and Donna Sousa to see their son, Ed, Jr., be ordained as a priest in the Providence Rhode Island Diocese. When a priest is ordained, his hands are consecrated and anointed with the Oil Sacred Chrism and then wiped with a special linen cloth. The hands are anointed by the bishop's hands.

It was during this consecration that my eyes and heart opened more to my doubts about serving the Eucharist. The four men being ordained had radiant happiness on their faces. They waited at least seven years before finally receiving the honor to serve the Body and Blood of Christ to the parishioners. Their love for Jesus and Mary couldn't be mistaken by their constant smiles.

We are all human beings who have sins on our souls, including priests. But we don't have our hands anointed by bishops' hands for this sacred honor. In fact, I was astonished when there was absolutely no education or classes for me to take for such a responsibility.

It left me saddened not to hear anything about this important task. I sat in church with the other parishioners who signed for the ministry. The priest gave no sermon expressing the significance of serving. There was little training. We were only shown where to stand on the altar and instructed to fill in if a person was missing on their assigned Mass.

I learned from Father Ed, that Diocesan priests like him make promises, while religious order priests, such as the Franciscans and Dominicans, take vows. They give everything up in their life to serve God. It was a very emotional experience to witness the ordination. I felt the Holy Spirit during the whole Mass.

Father Ed served his first Mass and again Al, Arlene, and I attended, with pride, to witness the occasion. During Mass, the linen cloth the bishop had used to wipe Father Ed's hands during his ordination was placed around the hands of his mother. This cloth will then be bound around Donna's hands at her burial.

Father Ed had a spiritual bond with Nancy Latta from Medjugorje after she helped him in his decision for priesthood. The bishop allowed him another cloth for her. There had never been such a request. He felt his promises would not have been taken without Nancy's guidance over the past six years. Since he would not be there for their wedding anniversary, he made a trip to Medjugorje and presented it to Nancy a week before their actual date.

I was in worse turmoil mentally after sharing in Father Ed's special day. I was so confused on what I should do with this decision, until Al said to me, "If you feel this strong about your new belief not serving, then you shouldn't be serving at all."

I didn't sign up again for the ministry in June of 2005. My fellow ministers may not agree with me, but it was my decision to step down. The choice had been painful, because I knew every person who served with me on the altar, was a good, practicing Catholic. They have a powerful love for the Church and Jesus, as I do. In my heart and soul, I believe this holy honor belongs to the priests.

I had always been taught that serving the Holy Sacrifice of the Mass had to be reserved for males, so it would set an example and invitation, for young men to embrace the priesthood.

I do realize that some priests need help with serving Holy Communion, but there are Masses that have more than ten Eucharistic Ministers on the altar all at once. Another minister had told me that the main reason for this is because it would take too long to serve the parishioners.

When it did take awhile, it gave the people going down the aisle a chance to realize the holiness of what they were receiving and to ask for forgiveness for their sins. There was a time for prayers before rushing down the aisle to take Holy Communion.

When I had served, I had seen many parishioners, take the holy host and throw it into their mouth fast, with no expression of devotion. During my ministry, I'd been touched by one woman, who openly showed her true adoration for Jesus. When she stood in front of me to receive, she had uncontrollable tears coming down her face when she took the host on her tongue. The love on her face had said it all. I'd never forgotten that special and holy moment. God had let me witness what receiving His Body and Blood was meant to be.

For years, I've been taught that Communion was never to be handled by anyone receiving it. Parishioners had waited with eagerness for the priest to place the host onto our tongue, as we knelt at the altar rail.

It had been a blessed and divine honor to have received Jesus this way. I only pray we are not, innocently, abusing His sacred Body.

I personally miss the old traditions and practices in our church. There's fear within me seeing our Blessed Sacrament pushed to a side area of the altar. The Tabernacle is not a side shrine. In my heart, it belongs always in the CENTER of the altar. Isn't He the center of our lives? Is Satan chipping away at our religion hoping for us to fall into his trap?

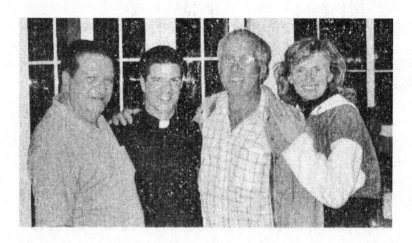

Left: Ed Sousa, Father Ed, Pat Latta & Nancy Latta

Father Ed's life story is covered in the 2003 Winter Medjugorje magazine on pages 40-43 Subscription: Medjugorje Magazine, PO Box 373, Westmont, IL 60559.

Chapter 55
The Miracle of Corey

On October 17, 2003, my daughter, Lori called me, in tears, when she and Mark rushed to the hospital to see their first grandchild's birth. This was Lori's second marriage and Mark's son's baby. The family was warned by the doctors that the chances of the baby being born alive were very slim: after a sonogram, they had discovered the lungs were undeveloped.

At the time, Lori had been struggling to find her faith. She had told me earlier that she wasn't even sure what she believed in. This was something I couldn't fathom, after bringing her and Debbie to church every Sunday. I had never wondered or questioned if my daughters believed in God. I automatically assumed Lori was a strong Catholic at heart, even though she didn't practice it. I had strayed, myself. I understood her separation from the church and did not want to judge her.

I try to pray the rosary everyday for my whole family to turn back to Jesus. I don't believe in pushing them. God gives all of us free will, so I keep my faith, that He will call them back. I have always offered my suffering (mentally and physically) up for them. Each day I consecrate their conversion up to the Sacred Heart of Jesus and the Immaculate Heart of Mary.

Lori was aware that my faith is solid. She begged me to put the baby on my prayer-line and to say a rosary. I explained how important it was for her to do the same. She wanted so much to believe as I did.

Without belief, we leave ourselves wide open for Satan to take over our souls. We lose our faith in God's mercy and miracles. Daily prayer connects us to Him and we learn to trust. Many gifts and graces are received keeping Jesus in our lives.

To the doctors' amazement, little Corey was born October 18, 2003. Another miracle Dad had talked about: when doctors gave no hope. Corey's lungs were fine, but his kidneys were not functioning normally. In 2005, they were supposed to start testing family members to see if one of them could become a kidney donor.

Chapter 56
Dedication of the WWII Memorial

In March of 2004, I heard that a memorial was going to be dedicated to the WWII veterans in Washington, D.C. on Memorial Day. I spoke to my brother, Joe, about it and he went on the website to register our father's name with the rank he had held at the time of WWII.

As time passed, I developed a strong desire to learn more about my father's life during the war. I went on the internet and searched for any information about WWII. I punched in Col. Albert L. Gramm, and to my complete shock, his name appeared with the mention of his unit, the 101st Infantry, 1st Battalion, Company B, of the 26th Yankee Division.

During the WWII battles, his duties progressively went from: Infantry Platoon Leader, Company Commander, Battalion Operations Officer S-3, Regimental S-3 Division Assistant G-3, the Battalion Commander, and Combined Arms Task Force Commander. He fought in the major battles in the Lorraine Campaign, Metz, along with the Battle of the Bulge.

The 26th Yankee Division went into full force after the Germans crashed throughout Europe in May 1940. America felt the need for increased defenses against the threat of totalitarian might, and started into operations long prepared plans for the mobilization of a citizen army. All nations National Guard Divisions were inducted into Federal Service within a year. And so, on January 16, 1941, the 26th Division, the "Yankee Division" of World War II, was inducted on that date, and the 10,000 Massachusetts Officers and men of the Division reported to the 50 Armories throughout the State.

Because of this threat, trainees were engaged in its initial training at Camp Edwards, Massachusetts to Fort Devens, Massachusetts for preliminary field maneuvers. The Regiment again moved to Camp Edwards in September 1941. They moved to participate in Carolina Maneuvers during October and November, returning again in December to Camp Edwards.

The world was stunned by the attack on Pearl Harbor on December 7, 1941. For the 26th Division, it meant immediate assignments to the Eastern Defense Command to aid in the security of the U.S.'s East Coast. The Regiment was engaged in shore patrol duty.

Training and preparations were completed in a year, and the Regiment moved to Camp Campbell, Kentucky, to Tennessee maneuvers, to Fort Jackson, South Carolina, and finally to Camp Shanks, New York. On September 7, 1944, the 101st Infantry Regiment docked in Cherbourg, France.

The Battle of the Bulge lasted December 16, 1944 to January 25, 1945. It was the largest Land Battle the U.S. Army has fought during World War II and to this date. **The Ardennes Offensive** (called **Operation Wacht Am Rhein** by the German Military Time), officially named the **Battle of the Ardennes** by the U.S. Army (and to the general public as the **Battle of the Bulge**).

The Battle of Ardennes was destined to be one of the fiercest and most trying of all for the 101st Infantry. More than a million men fought in this battle totaling 600,000 Germans, 500,000 Americans and 55,000 British.

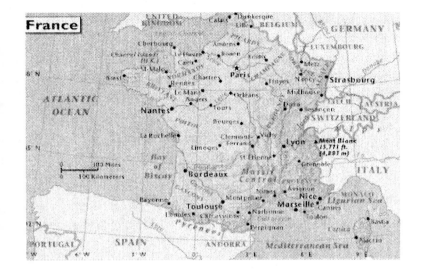

France and Germany borders
(Battle of Metz & Lorraine: upper right)

After receiving all this information, I placed an ad on site of the 26th Yankee Division, asking for any feedback from anyone who might have served alongside of him. Within weeks, I had received replies back from servicemen by e-mail, personal letters and phone calls. Veterans sent me their memorabilia that they had intended to save for their own families.

Colonel Leonid Kondratiuk, a retired director from the US Army, referred me to the recently published book *The Command is Forward; The 101st Infantry In Lorraine* written by James C. Haahr. In its narrative, my father was mentioned several times: on pages 93, 115 (twice) and 140. The book will be a treasured item to me because it mentions many of the locations where my father fought.

My father went to Camp Drum in New York for training. Fort Drum, its original name, was created in 1908 as Pine Camp, a 10,000-acre summer reserve training camp. From 1942-1944, a number of buildings were built for housing and training. During this period, a mobilization hospital was constructed in the old post 2400 area with capacity to house 540 patients. Medical facilities had been erected as a result of the rapid expansion during World War II. In 1951, Pine Camp was designated as Camp Drum. Certain portions of the hospital continued to be occupied to support the reserve training mission.

I continued to search the website for information on Camp Drum, when I came upon a Jim Neville, who was the Curator for Fort Drum Historical Collections. I emailed him and asked if there was any information on my father. He answered right away saying yes, and that he was trying to put a memorial together for the 26th Yankee Division. Jim wanted pictures of Dad and hoped to dedicate a private memorial for him. He informed me that very little information was ever gathered about the 26th Yankee Division during WWII so I sent him what my mother had gathered from her scrapbooks.

Jim wrote back to me, and through his record searching, he found that a WWII unit history, "26 Infantry Division-Yankee Division," published by Turner Publishing Company, mentions a Major Gramm in conjunction with the German surrender of the St. Jeanne d'Arc fortress outside of Metz, France, on December 13, 1944.

A Joe Devine of North Weymouth called to introduce himself. He and his brother Ed had served under my father. Ed had since passed away. He told me that in 1942, the company was divided into three parts: one third went to the Pacific and one third formed a new unit. He said it had to be a hard decision for my father to decide how to separate the men and split up the division.

Ed and Joe were assigned to the new unit, the 328th Infantry. My father fought to keep the two together for a while, but back then, the military did not want to keep brothers in the same unit during combat. There had been too many records of brothers dying together at the same location of a battle. Ed had solved the problem by joining a Parachute Unit shortly afterward.

Joe had written his memoirs for his family and was going to throw them away until he heard from me. He wrote, "You're an excellent salesperson!" They were published in his local newspaper. He stated that the night before the war ended, November 18, 1944, it was bitterly cold and snowed heavily until daybreak. Joe had lost all feelings in his feet and couldn't walk that morning. His medical team diagnosed him with Trench Foot.

He'd been hospitalized in England. Upon healing, his commanding officer asked him if he would return to the front. Joe told me, "I believe if it had been your father asking, I would've been unable to refuse. Remembering those days is a bittersweet experience, but be assured I'm happy to do what I can to keep the memory of your father alive."

A boy by the name of Jared replied by e-mail that he had just returned from a trip through the battlefields and sites of Luxembourg with his grandfather, Bernard Huntley. Bernard served in the same company as my father, from December to January. Jared had stood on the cemetery hill near Café Schumann where apparently large numbers of the unit had been gunned down. He and his grandfather had walked through the woods to the same foxholes the unit had occupied.

He was sure his grandfather couldn't remember my father because of the short length of time he was with them. Jared stated that the unit was hit particularly hard during the battle at Schumann's Eck and they had merged with another company. His grandfather had also caught Trench Foot. Jared wrote that Belgium and Luxembourg had not forgotten what our troops had gone for their countries.

Bernard Huntley replied back to me on his own and still frequently keeps in touch. He sent me pictures of my father to add to my collection. After Bernard completed his memoir, he sent me a full copy so I would have an idea of what the war was like for my father. It gave the true reactions and fear the men had had during the war.

Richard I. Paul of Destin, Florida sent me a letter, after seeing my ad in *Yankee Doings* magazine. He wanted to assure me that my father was well remembered by those who still survived. He'd been asked to give a speech about the 26th Infantry Yankee Division in combat during WWII, at the Crowne Plaza in Worcester. He confessed there were very few WWII Veteran in attendance.

Richard described my father as, "An outstanding battalion commander." He had had the opportunity to be with Dad in combat and said that he had performed his duties in a superior manner. Richard said he was a calm and competent officer. He enclosed a copy of his speech with his letter.

Dennis J. O'Brien, of Ft. Myers Beach, Florida, was a member of Company G of the 104th Infantry. He served in the National Guard from 1947 until retiring in 1989. Dennis remembered my father and said he was well liked by all the officers and enlisted men. He sent a picture of my father: down on the ground, showing the guardsman how to get into the proper position to fire their rifles. My father had worn military khakis instead of his officer's uniform that day.

Dennis said, "That was the kind of officer he was. He set an example for the rest to follow. Your dad was certainly a great asset to the National Guard and to the people that knew him. I'm glad to have known him personally."

Frederick N. Kawa of Whitman, Massachusetts, saw my inquiry in the *Yankee Doings*. He's still affiliated with the Army and served in the Air Force from 1965-1968. He fought in Vietnam in his last year of active duty. He had worked with Joe St. Onge, Joe Furtado, my brother Albert, and my father at Pyrotector, in Hingham. Dad's influence helped him get into the Army Officer Candidate program and he was commissioned in 1978. Today he is a retired Lieutenant Colonel.

All the replies that poured in made me realize what personal stories I had missed hearing directly from my father. My nephew, David, told me that Dad had often talked about the war with him. He probably had had the comfort to talk with David because he was his grandson. The difference was: David asked. He had showed his grandfather interest in his wartime years. Someday, I hope to hear those stories.

Years have passed: many deceased servicemen could've supplied me with important information about Dad's activities if I had asked and showed interest ten years sooner. Most of his close friends that had served along side him are gone. They had known him better than anyone else.

Leona believed Dad never would've opened up to me, even if I had asked. She said the only people he talked to about the war were his close Army friends. I saw the effect of the war when I met a veteran while Al and I were shopping in Dartmouth.

An elderly man, in his late eighties rode by me on his scooter in the store. He stopped and joked with me because he couldn't find his wife, who was somewhere in the store. I laughed and told him he was lucky to have wheels under him to search for her. Both of us had polite talk until I noticed his Navy cap on his head with a WWII pin on it.

I asked him about his service years. He mentioned that he had fought in Normandy and was in therapy because of the nightmares he still has. I tried to tell him how important it was for him to tell his stories to his family.

He told me, "In two hours, two thousand young men were dead on the beach. We had no idea where the enemy was when they were shooting at us. How'd you like to come upon arms and legs all over the place, or pick up a helmet, and see a head still in it?" Without any control, the man suddenly went into complete tears and started moving down the aisle in the store. I heard him repeatedly saying, over and over, as he wheeled away from me, "I just can't talk about it anymore!"

I stood there, feeling guilty to have brought up the war. It was so long ago! The effect on him made me realize that maybe Leona was right. Dad had probably felt the same way as that veteran—maybe worse, since he had been a commanding officer, watching his men die in front of him. He had to make major decisions for them.

Soldiers had been killed because that was the only way the rest stayed alive to come home. They came face to face with strangers who would instantly become their enemies. Many young boys held rifles, each wanting to live as much as the next. Wars are not between people—they are between countries. It's all political.

No matter what war our men and women have fought in, the faces of those they've killed, must be embedded in their minds. Watching someone suffer and die in front of you has to be mentally devastating. It's sad, because no one wants to be there in the first place.

No wonder Dad was afraid to go to confession. He had defended his country and lived with the fear that God would not forgive him. Veterans need to believe God is merciful.

The WWII Memorial was dedicated to the veterans in Washington, D.C. on Memorial Day May 31, 2004. Dad would've been so proud to be a part of the tribute. Who knows, maybe he was there in spirit. After hearing that Our Lady allowed one of the visionaries to see and talk to her mother after her death, anything is possible.

The Gramm family is honored to have our father listed in the WWII Memorial Book along with the other men and women who fought in WWII. Someday family members hope to travel to Washington, D.C. and embrace the recognition finally given to the WWII veterans.

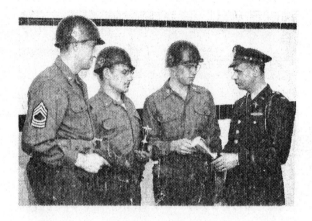

Dad on Right: Receiving a Rifle Award

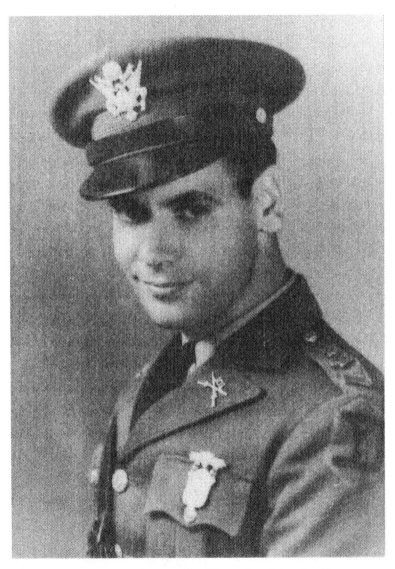

Brigadier General, Albert L. Gramm, Sr.

Chapter 57
A New Addition

On Sunday, July 31, 2005 Joe and Marge flew to Guatemala to welcome and bring home their adopted daughter, Molly Jannette Gramm. She was born on March 9, 2005. The family was delighted with our new addition to the family. Dad has to be looking down from Heaven with a big smile and a heart full of love. God brings special children into our lives for reasons even beyond our own comprehension.

Our mother, at ninety-two years old, was able to witness and hold a new grandchild. What a blessing from God.

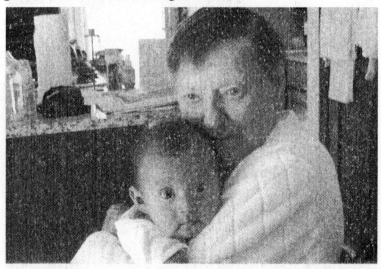

Molly and Mom

Chapter 58
A Faith Restored

After collecting pictures, written articles, and memorabilia of my father, I started to put it all together. Death had waited around the corner and took him when I least expected it. It's important to realize that our parents have so much to teach us. They're our history. In the past, they made the same mistakes we are making, but as children, we don't listen or take their advice on how to do things right.

So much time, energy, and sorrow could be saved if we were to pay attention to them. Our children think we, as parents, are old. They laugh at us, thinking we are outside the times, and what do we know? Children insist the world has changed since those *old days!* But morals and worshipping God are still the same as they have been since the beginning of time.

It was the parents who changed. Many of us are not teaching our children about faith and a living God. Children need to see their parents going to church and hear them talk openly about having trust and belief in Jesus. If we don't, they won't.

Individuals are intimidated easily and don't fight to keep our values for ourselves, families or schools. We are afraid to say the word God publicly or simply wish someone a *Merry Christmas.*

The courts, judges, politicians, school principles and many in authority have stepped back, knowing how bad some of the choices are that they make for us. No one dares to make a moral move on an issue.

The decision-makers are afraid of losing their positions in the next election year, so they do what they think is right for their careers. They too easily forget the fact that we vote them into office because of the promises they make to do what is best for the people, the communities and our country.

Anything that is involved around spirituality makes them freeze. Getting rid of religious topics as soon as possible, even if it means passing it to another person, takes the pressure off them. Yet, our fore fathers fought and died making decisions around their belief, faith and worship in God. They knew the importance of having Him in their lives, speech and documents. They gave us what we have today and now we want to erase it. Through the centuries, millions have been killed protecting the word of God so we could have religious freedom. God can't, and won't, be erased from this earth. It's His world, not ours.

One single person can change the whole judicial system by keeping God's name out of whatever they're trying to control. Many of us step back doing nothing about it. *How powerful is Satan?* Don't you think he has a hand in trying to remove God from everything? We are slowly allowing it to happen.

When I sat back and studied my life, I realized just how much my father had taught me about believing in God. The most important thing I've learned was to never stop worshiping. He had a lot of knowledge to pass down to the family. If he could say anything to us, I believe it would be to love one another.

Dad knows it all now. He's surrounded by only peace and love. The little things he had worried about on Earth are gone. I'm sure he now knows that material things should not have meant so much while he was alive.

Our fathers on Earth take the place of Our Father in Heaven, like St. Joseph did with Jesus. I believe that from birth, we are placed in a learning process until our death. God puts individuals in our path to lead us to Him. We have to watch and listen for their arrival. Like Dad said, "Take notice."

God wants all of us to share in His eternal happiness no matter how greatly we sin. We are given until our very last breath to choose between Our Savior or Satan. Our salvation will come from believing in His teachings to reach the Kingdom of Heaven. He reserves a place for every person from the day of our creation. It's up to us if we want it.

God does not judge so much on how many times we have sinned, rather how sorry we are in our hearts for committing the sins. That's why we have penance. God gave us Ten Commandments to follow as a ticket to Heaven.

Our days should start and end with Jesus in our hearts. We're always praying and asking for things but we need to thank Him when they're given to us. Most importantly, bring God to your children. It's our responsibility as parents to practice our faith with them. We're going to be held accountable for it at the end.

Forget what mistakes happened yesterday and don't worry about tomorrow. It's not here yet. Do one good deed for someone else each day that faces you. It could be as simple as giving a warm smile to a person who just took the only seat left on the bus. Now, that's a sacrifice! Offer any situation that's upsetting to you up for sinners or non-believers to convert. Never forget the Souls in Purgatory.

We should stop looking at all the negative things in our life. Look at the good. Our lives are surrounded by daily changes and they may disrupt things for awhile until the answers come to us. That's the time we need God the most.

In the book *My Imitation of Christ* by Thomas a'Kempis; the author states, "When Jesus is present, all things go well and nothing seems difficult, but when Jesus is absent, everything is hard. When Jesus speaks not within, our comfort is worthless, but when Jesus speaks within, we feel great consolation." God speaks to us in many different ways every day to lead us in the right direction, we just need to listen.

If life is always upside-down with no peace or happiness, stop and try to understand why. Believe it or not, a high percentage of our failures or hurt, come from us. Maybe it was from choosing the wrong mate, staying in a dull, boring job that went nowhere, hanging out with the wrong friends to be popular, or having children without planning parenthood.

We can feel sorry for ourselves, and blame God for all the bad things that happen, or we can start making good decisions in our lives. Before getting in a bad relationship or situation, stop and take notice to the signs. Does a partner make us feel good about ourselves? Are we happy with them? Are we treated with love? Are we uncomfortable with certain friends? If it doesn't seem right or good…it probably isn't. End it *fast*. That's where our free will comes into play.

As I stated before, any turmoil in our life is the work of the devil. Everyone's life will have suffering and trials. It's our choice that will determine the outcome.

When it comes to parents, try to understand them. Not all relationships are good between them and their children. Maybe you have a good reason for not seeing or talking to them. If they disappointed or hurt you in some way, break down the wall that's between you. If you can't, try to forgive and move on—even if it's without them. Hating and holding anger, can take a lot of energy out of us. Becoming a bitter person can hold us from enjoying life and our families as God intended.

Does it *really* matter who is right or wrong? Pride is a killer. Letting go is a healthy way of healing. Don't let it divide you. *"When you stand to pray, forgive anyone against whom you have a grievance, so that your heavenly Father may in turn forgive you your transgressions"* *(Mark 11:25)*. Satan doesn't want any existence of unity within a family.

What a gift, if walls could come down in families, and we started loving again. Roles change with the elderly. They become the children, and we are the adult. It can be difficult and depressing for a parent to suddenly need their children's help.

Aging can be cruel to a once active mind and body. We are all going to get old, if God allows us to live that long. When my mother was eighty-three years old, she said, "I still feel the same in heart as I did at seventeen; it's my body that wouldn't move for me to enjoy doing the things that use to give me pleasure."

Care for them in their last days. We may be the last ones they see before leaving this world. Let it be with a smile and a warm hand, surrounded by family members that love them.

My father was right about miracles being all around me. I never took the time to look for them or even became aware of them happening. Since he has left this world and time has passed, I've come to see and learn why they went unnoticed.

God hadn't been in my heart and I omitted daily prayer. He would only enter my mind when something bad happened. If I didn't get what I wanted, when it was needed, or my way, I lost faith. I would never freely put my life into His hands and wait for His will. God knocks and we have to open the door.

He needs to become the air we breathe and be part of our every day life, not just when we need Him. The love from God is beyond our human imaginations.

Our Blessed Mother has been sent by Jesus for years to try to get our attention. We can't just sit there and say I believe, and it ends there. We have to pray, do penance, and go back to church.

Our Lady has stated to all the visionaries that Satan will no longer reign. There will be no more sin. If the world was going to end, I doubt if the visionaries would be having children. God will decide who stays or goes from the decisions we made after hearing all the warnings. The decision factor will be who ignored and denied Jesus, and who has loved and worshipped Him.

Our Lady will be leaving a permanent sign on Apparition Hill once the last visionary receives their tenth secret. They were told it'll be seen, but no one will be able to touch it and that there'll be no doubt on Earth, even from the unbelievers, that she was with us. Everyone around the world will be aware of this sign. We'll not have much time to convert after the chastisements begin. If you wait, it'll be too late. These are not my predictions but those which Our Lady tells the visionaries to pass on to us.

Converting can be as easy as changing ourselves by being patient when someone irritates us, accepting a person who may be different, forgiving someone who hurt us, or opening our eyes to the significance of giving a helping hand to another person in need. Always remember: look into a person's eyes, and see Jesus. Would you help Him?

The most important act of conversion is turning to daily prayer and going to church. Once we bring Jesus into our lives, we can then see the things happening around us, like the miracles my father described to me. That's when we have the Holy Spirit in us.

Pope John Paul II so often stated to the crowd, "Do not be afraid...Never doubt...Never tire." Prayer is such a simple thing. Don't give up on it and Jesus will bring the peace you're searching for in your life. It may not be the way you want, but it'll arrive. You just need faith. Give up the television and video games and take time to pray, especially as a family. Spend time together instead of everyone going their own ways.

During Dad's illness and death, Our Lord allowed me to suffer the pain of loss so I could learn from it. We'll never get over losing a loved one but we should find the faith to trust in God that they are safely home. Suffering is a gift to share with God and it should be offered up with love.

The miracle I had prayed for, for my father to stay with me longer, didn't come. God had plans for him. The reasons are far beyond me until we are reunited. I can't be selfish: he did live to be eighty years old and we still have our mother. Dad was a loving father who put his whole heart around his five children. I couldn't avoid his death but I had choices on how to deal with it. I pulled God back into my life and He's bringing me peace.

Don't stop praying because of the pain. He'll bring you comfort. *"Blessed are those who mourn, for they will be comforted" (Matthew 5:4).* Pray to Our Blessed Mother who knows your pain after watching her only Son die in agony from being tortured. He died still loving each and every one of us, despite all our rejections and sins.

A loved one leaves many memorable things for us with their passing. It may be one small thing, but it's a souvenir to hold onto. I kept a green and white plaid shirt of Dad's, which I wear while cleaning the house. Mom had given me his over-size rocking chair. What a treasure. It holds so many memories. I cherish a chipped plastic statue of the Pieta which sat on his bedside while he was dying.

When I looked at it during his illness, I imagined Our Lady holding him like Jesus. It reminded me of Jesus' remark to his mother when he was dying on the cross, *"Women, behold thy son. Son, behold thy mother" (St. John, 19.26).* We're all her children and she's our Heavenly Mother.

Take the time to talk to your parents and ask the questions that you hold in your heart before God takes them. The time is now. Ask them if they were happy in life, what were they like as children, what did they dream, what disappointments did they have, or did they miss out on something? Learn what they have to teach you.

Go beyond the material things. It had been a painful and heartbreaking experience for me to spend the last two weeks with my father. During his passing, doors opened for me to see the things he and God were trying to teach me about life and death. Our Lady called me to Medjugorje and she and Jesus gave me the healing I needed. It had been a beautiful journey in mind and soul.

My spiritual experiences are now treasured. My eyes and ears are more open to the miracles in my daily path since Dad passed away. We all belong to Jesus, and at the end, Our Savior calls us home.

My father left me with many gifts. They're indiscernible to others, but they were many. He was my gift from God. Through prayer, love, and faith, I let go knowing that someday I will be with him again.